Praise for *The Meals to Heal Cookbook*

"Susan Bratton and Jessica Iannotta have created a wonderful resource for anyone affected by cancer, and who is faced with the question, 'what should I eat?' *The Meals to Heal Cookbook* provides practical advice to address a variety of symptoms, plus plenty of information about what you can eat before, during, and after treatment to foster optimal health and well-being."

—Suzanne Dixon, MPH, MS, RDN, Epidemiologist and Registered Dietitian, Nutritionist, The Health Geek, LLC, Portland, Oregon

"In 2005, my mother was diagnosed with pancreatic cancer; my life changed after that day. Thanks to tireless effort from her doctors and a healthy lifestyle while receiving treatment she was able to fight her battle for over 9 years. From the very beginning of her battle my family and I knew that proper nutrition was a vital part of this fight. *The Meals to Heal Cookbook* brings proper nutrition to cancer patients in a way that is approachable—easy recipes that you don't need a culinary degree to prepare. My mother always knew how to bring joy and comfort to her loved ones and strangers as well. So in her honor I continue on her fight by doing all I can as a culinary professional to help those in need while fighting pancreatic cancer."

—Michael Ferraro, Executive Chef, Partner, Delicatessen, NY, NY

"Cancer survivors need resources to help them eat healthy during and after treatment. This cookbook is a wonderful resource which will no doubt introduce users to many new healthy foods that are easy to prepare. I look forward to trying many of these recipes myself! Thank you Susan and Jessica for giving us this cookbook to recommend to our patients!"

—Carolyn Lammersfeld, MS, RD, CSO, LD, MBA, VP Integrative Oncology, Cancer Treatment Centers of America

the meals to heal cookbook

From Savor Health: The Experts in Cancer Nutrition

the
meals to heal
cookbook

150 easy, nutritionally balanced recipes to nourish you during your fight with cancer

Susan Bratton and Jessica Iannotta,
MS, RD, CSO, CDN

Da Capo
LIFE LONG

A Member of the Perseus Books Group

Designed by Jack Lenzo
Set in 10.5 point Warnock by the Perseus Books Group

Library of Congress Cataloging-in-Publication Data
Names: Bratton, Susan (Food company executive) | Iannotta, Jessica.
Title: The Meals to Heal cookbook : 150 easy, nutritionally balanced recipes
   to nourish you during your fight with cancer / Susan Bratton and Jessica
   Iannotta, MS, RD, CSO, CDN.
Description: First Da Capo Press edition. | Boston, MA : Da Capo Lifelong
   Books, a member of the Perseus Books Group, 2016. | Includes
   bibliographical references and index. | Description based on print version
   record and CIP data provided by publisher; resource not viewed.
Identifiers: LCCN 2015047907 (print) | LCCN 2015044942 (ebook) | ISBN
   9780738218809 (e-book) | ISBN 9780738218793 (paperback) | ISBN
   9780738218809 (e-book)
Subjects: LCSH: Cancer--Diet therapy--Recipes. | Cancer--Patients--Nutrition.
   | BISAC: COOKING / Health & Healing / Cancer. | COOKING / Health & Healing
   / General. | LCGFT: Cookbooks.
Classification: LCC RC271.D52 (print) | LCC RC271.D52 B72 2016 (ebook) | DDC
   641.5/631--dc23
LC record available at http://lccn.loc.gov/2015047907

First Da Capo Press edition 2016

Published by Da Capo Press
A Member of the Perseus Books Group
www.dacapopress.com

Da Capo Press books are available at special discounts for bulk purchases in the U.S. by corporations, institutions, and other organizations. For more information, please contact the Special Markets Department at the Perseus Books Group, 2300 Chestnut Street, Suite 200, Philadelphia, PA, 19103, or call (800) 810–4145, ext. 5000, or e-mail special.markets@perseusbooks.com.

10 9 8 7 6 5 4 3 2 1

This book is dedicated to all those who have battled cancer as a patient or as someone who loves a patient with cancer. In particular, to Eric Stamp and his family, who inspired me to start Savor Health and devote the rest of my life to making proper nutrition something that is easily accessible and affordable to cancer patients and their families and that is supported and promoted by the medical industry.

And to my father, Dick Bratton, who won his battle with cancer against all odds. And to all of the amazing and inspirational patients and caregivers I have had the honor to work with over the past fifteen years. You inspire me every day to continue to make a difference in the lives of cancer patients—and through this book, to have the ability to touch the lives and reach even more patients and caregivers than I could have ever imagined.

Contents

Introduction

In the fall of 2008, I received a panicked call from my dear friend Eric. For some unknown reason, he explained, half of his face had collapsed, and he had been in the hospital for two days while doctors frantically searched for a diagnosis. He had just gotten the answer to the mystery: Eric was diagnosed with a glioblastoma of the brain stem—in other words, brain cancer. Although this diagnosis was devastating, Eric, an energetic and attractive man with a zest for life, responded with his usual optimism and started planning a trip to Germany for Oktoberfest the following year. But Eric's cancer quickly began to weaken him, and he struggled with debilitating symptoms.

Soon after his diagnosis, Eric's motor skills declined to the point where he could barely swallow or speak clearly, a consequence of the tumor's impacting his swallowing muscles. During this period, he received little direction from his health-care team about how and what to eat to help maintain his weight and optimal health throughout treatment, or to help reduce the severe side effects he was experiencing, particularly painful mouth sores and difficulty swallowing. In fact, he was told it didn't matter. His parents and brother searched for solutions, only to find that nothing legitimate existed. There were websites that contained nonscientific, often dangerous, information and recommendations as well as "legitimate" sites that actually contradicted one another's recommendations. Even then, these "legitimate sources" provided minimal actionable information. There was no single "go-to" source that offered comprehensible suggestions and recommendations that were also safe and based on scientific research. It was confusing, overwhelming, and frightening. As I watched him waste away and lose his ability to eat, and watched his family search for solutions, afraid to make a "wrong" decision, I couldn't help but think that there must be a way to make their lives easier and less stressful by avoiding or managing, if not the disease itself, at least these painful side effects and nutritional issues.

Eric ultimately lived only five months after his diagnosis, and his illness opened my eyes to an important and unmet health-care need. Cancer patients and caregivers all over the world, just like Eric and his family, need help managing and solving their nutritional issues during their treatment and survivorship. If they are too tired to cook, this help could be providing nutritious meals delivered to their home. If they are able to cook but still too tired to shop for groceries, it could simply be providing recipes. If they just want to talk to someone who is trained in oncology nutrition, it could be arranging for a phone call with this trained professional. Eric's and his family's struggle with nutrition is a common experience with cancer patients and cancer caregivers. It became clear to me that cancer patients and cancer caregivers need resources that empower them with helpful and safe information and services to take control of the one variable under their control: nutrition and food.

I was perplexed by the fact that few resources existed for Eric and his family, and that nutrition was not considered integral to his cancer treatment regimen. So, I took to researching on my own, seeking evidence-based findings on nutrition and the cancer patient. I spent the next year reading everything I could get my hands on, focusing on the role nutrition plays in the development and growth of cancer as well as on how nutrition and nutritional interventions can help cancer patients become or remain strong during treatment. As I immersed myself in the medical literature, I spoke with many cancer specialists, including doctors, nurses, social workers, and dietitians. I volunteered at Memorial Sloan Kettering Cancer Center, helping pediatric patients and their parents. I also attended a number of oncology conferences. From my research and in-person work with patients and their families, I learned that cancer treatment and disease-related side effects—including fatigue, lack of energy, mouth sores, difficulty swallowing, nausea, and vomiting—are a major impediment preventing cancer patients from eating and remaining well nourished. These side effects can also greatly diminish a patient's quality of life and mealtime enjoyment. I also found out that certain foods, ingredients, and meal preparations can prevent and mitigate side effects and, in doing so, prevent, slow, and even reverse malnutrition, not to mention make patients feel better, have more energy, and be able to enjoy life.

Good nutrition may not be able to cure cancer, but it can certainly provide supportive benefits and improve patients' well-being. The more I learned about the importance of proper nutrition and the difficulties that patients and caregivers experience with receiving proper nutrition and guidance, the more committed I became to helping people like Eric and his family find the resources they need.

I started Savor Health in 2011. Jessica Iannotta, a registered dietitian and certified specialist in oncology nutrition, joined me soon thereafter, and together, we have built Savor Health into what it is today. Savor Health provides solutions to the nutritional issues confronted by cancer patients and their families—access to healthy, nutritious home-delivered meals that are customized, using a proprietary technology platform, to help manage and mitigate specific side effects; oncology-trained dietitians who provide nutrition counseling; and approachable, evidence-based information and resources that help patients navigate the overwhelming world of cancer nutrition. What we have learned is that meals and recipes can be customized to help address the common side effects experienced by patients; our patients have benefited from recipes that are designed to manage their side effects telling us that our meals gave them more energy and reduced their side effects. A brain tumor patient who was a Savor Health customer for nearly one year told us that he looked forward to our healthy meals every week and they strengthened him in his fight and reduced his side effects. In another instance a group of breast cancer patients found that Savor Health's meals helped them to achieve and maintain a healthy weight during and after cancer treatment. This cookbook is part of our mission to provide both patients and caregivers healthy, easy to prepare recipes that not only taste delicious to both patients and their caregivers but also address the many side effects they experience. All of us at Savor Health hope that you enjoy these recipes, that they strengthen you during your cancer treatment and into survivorship, and that you find some joy in preparing meals and sharing mealtime together with your entire family.

Bon appétit!

Part 1

Getting Started

Food Can Change Your Cancer Journey

Eat food. Not too much. Mostly plants.

—Michael Pollan

More and more research is being done that validates the importance of eating real food and of eating plant-based foods. *Real food* means food that is not processed or preprepared in a package; it is essential that we eat foods in their whole, natural form. This means that cooking from scratch, using healthful, natural ingredients, is much healthier than preparing from a box. Real food focuses on whole fruits and vegetables, grains, legumes, nuts, dairy, fish, meat, and poultry that is eaten as is or prepared in a wholesome meal. With real foods, you know everything that is going into your meals, and that means no preservatives, additives, or artificial ingredients. Eating real food can also be much friendlier to your wallet—it is much less expensive than buying prepared food. Our emphasis is on real-food recipes that are easy to prepare so you can stay well nourished and maintain optimal health. From that underlying philosophy, our oncology-credentialed registered dietitians designed each recipe with cancer patients in mind, taking into account their unique nutritional needs.

Why These Recipes Are Beneficial for Cancer Patients

The most common nutritional issues for cancer patients include malnutrition, fatigue, and such side effects as lack of appetite, taste changes, mouth sores, and difficulty chewing and swallowing. Our team of oncology-credentialed registered dietitians focus on these common issues to help address and manage side effects so that eating is less stressful, more convenient, and simply more enjoyable, while still making sure each dish is nutritionally adequate. In addition, we provide recipe indexes for each side effect to help you find foods that you can tolerate during and after cancer treatment. Lastly, the recipes were designed with the entire family in mind so that even though you are ill, you can still enjoy mealtime with your family and enjoy the same dishes.

They Are Healthy and Nutritious

With growing information regarding the link between cancer (prevention, treatment, and survival) and nutrition, it is important to eat nutrient-rich foods rather than calorie-rich foods. The majority of our recipes have a plant-based and vegetarian foundation, as research shows eating a predominantly plant-based diet has many health benefits. All recipes were designed first and foremost from this nutritional perspective—they are well balanced with vital nutrients and provide a healthful amount of calories. Many of the recipes include tips on how to add more protein from plant or animal sources as well as information on how to adapt for varying side effects and symptoms. The portion size of each recipe in this book is manageable and appropriate for the majority of cancer patients and caregivers. For those who need to add calories, certain recipes tell you how to do so in a healthy way. You will not find any artificial ingredients here. You will, however, find satisfying, mostly plant-based dishes that ensure you get all of the fruits, vegetables, and protein for a healthy and strong *you*.

They Taste Good

Sometimes, getting adequate nutrition means exploring healthy foods that you may not have tasted or heard about before. Familiarizing yourself with a new food is not always easy, whether it be smooth, creamy lentils; bright, crunchy kale; or soft, fluffy quinoa, so we tried to make this journey a bit easier by collecting tempting, inviting recipes that use these ingredients. Knowing that taste issues are common among cancer patients, our recipes were also designed to be mouthwatering but still fall along a broad spectrum of flavor to meet a wide range of needs; many dishes are customizable so you can adapt flavors to suit common symptoms and make the most of each recipe without overwhelming your palate. You may have always enjoyed spicy food and loved meals like tacos, but with treatment have found that those flavors are harder to tolerate. These dishes were curated by our team of oncology-credentialed registered dietitians with flavor changes in mind—just because you can't handle the spice right now does not mean you need to do away with the tacos (just try our Tacos with Peppery Tomato Simmered Lentils [page 87]). Some of the recipes suggest adding hot pepper or hot sauce to the dishes for a little extra flavor in the event you've lost your sense of taste. Remember, you can always omit or substitute with a more welcoming spice.

They Are Easy to Chew, Swallow, and Digest

Because mouth sores, difficulty swallowing, or indigestion can be a common side effect of many cancer treatments, we paid special attention to ensure that our recipes are easy to chew, swallow, and digest. The majority of the recipes in this cookbook do *not* have crunchy, hard, or sticky textures. The dishes are easy to eat for a patient with very strong symptoms while still keeping an appealing mouthfeel and palate for those patients with minimal symptoms. For those with more bothersome digestive symptoms, we categorized our recipes to highlight the most tolerable ones. In addition, we provide suggestions and special tips in many of our recipes for how to adapt for enhanced digestive tolerance.

They Are Easy to Prepare

We know that not everyone is a master chef and we also know that some people love to cook. We also understand that whether you are a patient or a caregiver, you may not have the time or energy to prepare an elaborate meal. Each recipe provides the approximate preparation and cooking time; most can be prepared in thirty minutes or less. Some are easy to follow and very quick to prepare (the Frozen Banana Strawberry Bowls [page 198], just require a freezer and a blender). Of course, there are a few recipes that require some more time (such as those that need to be simmered or baked, like the Whole Wheat Chocolate Raisin Zucchini Bread [page 168], the Apple Crumble Baked Oatmeal [page 29], and the Broccoli Kale Lasagne [page 115]) and may require some more skill (such as the Grilled Beet and Goat Cheese Burgers [page 128], and the Chickpea Flour Pizza Margherita [page 132]), but you can work up to those and with time feel comfortable coming up with your own twists to these delicious and healthy meals.

How to Use This Book

Nutrition is such a critical component of your cancer journey and in maintaining strength during treatment. Our goal is to make it easy to accomplish nutritional health by providing you with information that will empower you to take control.

Many cancer patients are impacted by a variety of side effects that make it difficult, and often unpleasant, to eat and remain well nourished during cancer and cancer treatment, so look at the "Tips for Managing Side Effects" section (page 8) for some helpful information on managing and mitigating these. Check the list of "Noteworthy Ingredients" (page 14) to help familiarize you with the healthful whole foods these recipes use. We also review our top kitchen tools in the "Essential Kitchen Equipment and Cookware" section (page 24).

All recipes were developed with the help of oncology registered dietitians. These are professionals who have at least two thousand clinical hours of oncology dietetics, as well as successful completion of a national exam testing their proficiency in this area. So, you can be sure that each recipe has been developed with the very specific needs of cancer patients in mind. Throughout the book, look for the "CSO's Favorite to Savor" blurbs for special recipe highlights and nutrition tips.

There is so much confusing information out there about nutrition and oftentimes it is even contradictory. In the back of the book, we include a section titled "Information on Common Nutrition Topics" that you may reference. Because the immune system of a cancer patient can be more susceptible to infection, including that from food, we have a section discussing food safety and how to maintain a safe and healthy kitchen.

At the end of the book, two recipe indexes make recipe selection effortless and specific to your needs. Recipes by Side Effects and Symptoms (page 240) is a full list of the recipes organized by chapter and lists the symptoms that each recipe can address. This is a great starting place to begin searching for recipes that will help you manage your side effects and make it easier to eat and take in the nutrients that will strengthen you for your fight.

If you prefer to select recipes by symptom instead, we also include Top Recipes by Symptoms (page 251), which lists the common side effects experienced by cancer patients and the best recipes in this cookbook that are suited to help manage that specific side effect. So, however you like to think about cooking and meal preparation, we designed this cookbook to meet your needs.

To make recipe selection easy, each recipe features a list of what side effects it is best suited to help manage. For instance, in the example to the right, side effects marked with a plus sign (+) indicate that this recipe could help manage that particular side effect. If you are looking for quick meals, there is a special icon (⏱) that identifies the recipes that take 30 minutes or less to prepare.

Lack of Appetite	+
Nausea, Vomiting, or Heartburn	
Constipation	+
Diarrhea	
Fatigue	+
Mouth Sores	+
Dry Mouth	+
Chewing or Swallowing Difficulty	+
Taste Aversion— Sweet	
Taste Aversion— Sour & Bitter	
Lack of Taste	+
Smells Bother	+

Tips for Managing Side Effects

Cancer treatment can cause a variety of nutrition-related side effects. Many of these can be managed with changes in diet, appropriate food selection, and preparation. Following are some suggestions to help manage some of the common side effects and symptoms experienced during cancer treatment. Note that these suggestions are not a replacement for medical advice. Be sure to speak with your health-care team if you have persistent and bothersome symptoms that impact your ability to eat normally or maintain your weight.

Loss of Appetite: You may eat less than usual, not feel hungry at all, or feel full after eating only a small amount. Although you may not feel like eating, getting adequate nutrition and maintaining a healthy weight are important. Take advantage of the times when your appetite is strongest and try to consume small frequent meals and snacks throughout the day, such as the Blueberry Green Nut Butter Smoothie (page 171), the Classic Avocado Toast (page 46), or the Carrot Ginger Soup with Cashew Cream (page 155). Try to eat in enjoyable surroundings and make meals look less overwhelming by placing them on smaller rather than larger plates.

Nausea and Vomiting: Some types of chemotherapy can cause nausea and vomiting. Nausea is sometimes described as an unsettling or queasy feeling in the stomach and can be experienced with or without vomiting. Because an empty stomach may make nausea and vomiting worse, be sure to eat regular meals and snacks. Eat small, frequent meals (five or six times a day) instead of three large meals, and avoid greasy or spicy foods and food with strong odors. Eat dry foods, such as crackers, toast, and pretzels, which may be easier on your stomach. Try ginger teas, ginger candies, or gingersnaps or cookies, or add fresh ginger to soups and stir-fries. Our favorite recipes for soothing symptoms of nausea and vomiting include the Ginger Granita (page 209) and the Vegetable Chicken Soup (page 162).

Fatigue: This common side effect is usually described as feeling very weak, tired, or having a lack of energy. Choose foods high in protein and calories, which provide lots of energy, such as our Sweet Potato, Tomato, and Spinach Hash (page 59) and our Fudgy Date and Almond Truffles (page 196). The body is made up of about 70 percent water, so make sure to stay hydrated to keep your body running. Also try to incorporate some physical activity into your day, as studies have shown that exercise can boost mood and increase energy levels. Exercise may also help you gain an appetite. For a great energy boost, try our Vanilla Almond Chia Seed Shake (page 175) or our Avocado Mango Smoothie (page 170). Smoothies are a great way to get a lot of nutrition in just a few sips.

Constipation: Constipation can be caused by certain chemotherapies, nausea and pain medications, a change in diet, or a decrease in your usual activity level. Be sure to stay hydrated by drinking at least eight to ten 8-ounce glasses of fluid each day. Eat foods rich in fiber, such as fresh fruits and vegetables, beans, nuts, whole grains, and bran. The Thai-Style Vegetable Strand Salad (page 71), Multi-Bran Sour Cream Muffins (page 44), and Hearty Tomato Lentil Soup (page 153) are three of our top recipes for combating constipation.

Diarrhea: Diarrhea occurs when you experience frequent, loose, soft, or watery bowel movements, and it can quickly lead to dehydration. To minimize diarrhea, avoid greasy or fatty food, food high in fiber, raw vegetables, and caffeine. Drink a minimum of eight to ten 8-ounce glasses of clear fluid a day, such as water, broth, juice, ice pops, or decaffeinated tea. Consume foods rich in potassium, such as bananas and potatoes (without skin). Also eat foods high in pectin and soluble fiber, such as applesauce, baked apples, bananas, rice, and oatmeal to help slow down diarrhea. The Sweet or Savory Matzoh Brei (page 54), the Sweet Baked Banana Oatmeal (page 30), and the Roasted Applesauce (page 167) may feel soothing on an upset stomach.

Changes in Taste and Taste Aversion: Often during treatment, the foods you usually like can become unappealing. Foods may taste bland, bitter, or metallic. Try rinsing with 1 to 2 ounces of baking soda rinse before and after meals (recipe for baking soda rinse: 1 quart of water, ¾ teaspoon of salt, and 1 teaspoon of baking soda). If red meats taste strange, try substituting other proteins, such as chicken, turkey, fish, eggs, dairy, beans, or tofu. Eat foods that smell and look good to you. Avoid using metal utensils; use plastic ones instead. Avoid hot foods to reduce strong odors; serve food at room temperature instead.

Certain "flavor fixes" can also help to make a meal more tolerable. For example, if you are experiencing a metallic taste, flavor foods with onion, garlic, basil, oregano, rosemary, tarragon, mint, ketchup, barbecue sauce, or mustard. If foods taste too sweet, add six drops of lemon or lime juice, or until the sweet taste is muted. If foods are too salty, add ¼ teaspoon of lemon juice or sweeten foods with syrup, honey, or a pinch of sugar. If foods are too bitter or sour, add a little sweetener, such as maple syrup, honey, or a pinch of sugar. If foods taste like cardboard, add sea salt or a spritz of lemon or lime juice, or vinegar.

If you have an aversion to sweet foods, focus on more savory dishes, such as the Lemony Chickpeas with Parsley (page 81), the Roasted Vegetable Tostadas (page 86), or the Southwestern Veggie Burgers with Avocado Cilantro Mayo (page 130). If you have an aversion to sour or bitter foods, focus on sweeter options, such as the Eggless Banana Battered French Toast (page 42), the Chicken, Apple, and Maple Breakfast Patties (page 65), or the Whipped Sweet Potato Pie (page 208).

Mouth Soreness: Many patients treated with high-dose chemotherapy drugs and radiation treatment to the head and neck area can develop mucositis and mouth soreness. Avoid acidic and spicy foods along with rough and coarse foods that can irritate the oral cavity. It is helpful to eat nutrient-dense, soft foods, such as creamed soups, broth, pudding, scrambled eggs, yogurt, mashed potatoes, cottage cheese, shakes, smoothies, and nutritional drinks. Sometimes a straw can divert liquids away from painful areas. Some people may require prescription-numbing rinses before mealtime to reduce pain. Try the Cool Cucumber Avocado Soup (page 149), the Sweet Potato and Broccoli Mac and Cheese (page 105), or the Secret Ingredient Chocolate Avocado Fudgsicles (page 204) to help cool you down while still giving you a big nutritional boost.

Dehydration: Adequate fluids are important to prevent dehydration and to help your body function optimally. Many people are required to drink at least eight to ten 8-ounce glasses of fluid daily and urinate frequently during the first 24 hours after treatment to help flush the chemotherapy out of the kidneys. Sources of fluids include water, decaffeinated tea, juices, broths, fruit ices, ice pops, and gelatin. If you are finding it hard to drink plain water to maintain hydration, you can try flavoring it with different combinations of your favorite flavors of lime, lemon, orange, kiwi, watermelon, strawberry, green apple, cucumber, mint, rosemary, or ginger.

Heartburn and Reflux: Heartburn can be a side effect of chemotherapy. To minimize this, avoid acidic foods like tomatoes and citrus, strong flavors like mint and chocolate, as well as high-fat and spicy foods. Small frequent meals, and sipping fluids between meals rather than with meals, avoiding tight-fitting clothing, and not lying down too soon after mealtime can minimize acid regurgitation and discomfort. Some people may require over-the-counter or prescription acid-blocking medications recommended by their health-care team. If you're looking for recipes to manage heartburn, try our Simple Mushroom Soup (page 156) or Panfried Tofu and Vegetables over Brown Rice (page 138).

Food Safety "Best Practices"

Safe food handling is important for all cancer patients. Cancer treatments can weaken the immune system, making one more susceptible to infection, including that from food.

Certain foods are more likely to contain harmful bacteria and are considered higher risk for a cancer patient. These foods (and foods that include these items as an ingredient) should be avoided in those patients currently undergoing treatment. These include:

- Raw or undercooked eggs (including over-easy, poached, soft-boiled, and sunny-side up eggs)
- Foods made with uncooked eggs, such as salad dressings, raw cookie dough, and homemade eggnog
- Raw or undercooked meat and poultry
- Game meats
- Raw or undercooked fish, including sushi, sashimi, cold smoked or pickled fish or lox
- Hot dogs and luncheon meats that have not been reheated
- Unpasteurized milk, cheese, and juice
- Aged and veined cheeses, such as blue cheese or Roquefort (also including salad dressings containing these cheeses)
- Raw milk or unpasteurized versions of cheeses, including Brie, Camembert, and queso fresco (also including salad dressings containing these cheeses)
- Raw alfalfa sprouts and radish sprouts
- Unwashed fruits and vegetables and store-bought meals containing potentially unwashed items
- Foods made with miso or miso paste (fermented soy paste)
- Cereals, grains, nuts, seeds, or dried fruits purchased from a bulk bin

Following, we address some ingredients that are higher in risk and give you an excellent option for a safer ingredient.

Cheese: Soft cheeses made from unpasteurized milk, such as feta, Brie, Camembert, and queso fresco and aged blue-veined cheeses are a higher risk ingredient because they may be made from raw milk that is not pasteurized or may go through an extra aging process. Instead, it is safest to opt for cream cheese, cottage cheese, mozzarella, processed cheeses, and soft cheeses clearly labeled "from pasteurized milk," which are a lower risk for a cancer patient.

Eggs: Foods that contain raw or undercooked eggs, such as Caesar salad dressing, homemade raw cookie dough, or entrées that contain poached or sunny-side up eggs put those with a compromised immune system more at risk. Some recipes in this book use eggs in various forms. Since our cookbook can also be used by cancer survivors and caregivers, please use your discretion when choosing the best form of egg that is right for you and pay attention to the notes in each recipe for those with compromised immune systems. To be safe, choose pasteurized eggs and egg products, always keep eggs refrigerated, and discard any cracked eggs. Try hard-boiling or scrambling eggs for a safe alternative, or do a hard-poach.

If you are not currently undergoing treatments or if you are a cancer survivor, caregiver, or family member and are generally healthy, you may decide that the low risk of getting food borne illness is worth the pleasure of eating runny eggs. Again, be sure to purchase pasteurized eggs, always keep your eggs refrigerated, and discard eggs with any cracks. Some of our recipes call for a poached egg or runny yolk as an addition to or part of a recipe. If you want to be extra safe, you can always substitute a different style of egg or cook the yolk until completely firm. Be sure to check with your health-care team about the foods that are safe for you to eat.

Following is a list of recipes in this book that call for a runny egg. If you are currently undergoing cancer treatment and/or have a compromised immune system, fully cook the egg until the yolk is firm.

- Bull's-Eye Skillet Avocado Eggs (page 47)
- Red and Green Eggs Florentine (page 49)
- Cracked Eggs in Zucchini-Corn-Lime Sauté (page 55)
- Sweet Potato, Tomato, and Spinach Hash (page 59)
- Seitan, Apple, and Broccoli Breakfast Hash (page 62)

Noteworthy Ingredients

Here we highlight some noteworthy ingredients that are the foundation for many of our recipes in this cookbook. Some ingredients may be familiar, such as lentils, soy milk, and honey, while others may be new to you, such as chickpea flour, buckwheat groats, hemp milk, or agave nectar. Our go-to oil is olive oil for its versatile use and prominent staple of the Mediterranean diet, but we also like to experiment with other oils, such as coconut and safflower. This section also features a few of our favorite spices, such as turmeric and cardamom, not only for their exceptional flavors, but also for their disease-fighting properties. All the following ingredients can be part of a healthy diet. We encourage you to vary your diet, try new foods, and get cooking!

Plant-Based Proteins

Since this book emphasizes eating mostly vegetarian, plant-based foods because of their proven health benefits, we review the wide variety of plant-based foods that are rich in protein. Protein is important for maintaining strength and energy, and you can meet your daily needs by eating a mix of legumes, nuts, seeds, and soy.

LEGUMES

Dried beans are great to have on hand, and while they take a long time to cook, they are significantly cheaper than buying canned beans. Presoak the beans in water for at least 6 hours or overnight. Drain the beans, cover with at least an inch of water, bring to a boil, then lower the heat, cover the pot, and simmer for anywhere from 2 to 4 hours, stirring occasionally, until the beans are very tender. If you have a pressure cooker, you can cook beans much faster and more evenly, but a pot on the stove works just as well as long as you give it time.

Chickpea flour has fewer calories and carbohydrates than whole wheat or all-purpose flour and it packs in more protein. This flour is also a great source of folate, vitamin B_6, iron, magnesium, and potassium. Swap out half of the flour in a regular pancake recipe for chickpea flour, or try our Chickpea Flour Pizza Margherita (page 132).

Lentils are a great way to keep that savory texture without the added fat, calories, and cholesterol that come with meat. Lentils come in all kinds of beautiful colors, from red to yellow to green and brown, and they are high in fiber and iron. Try our Cheesy Lentil "Meatballs" (page 122) or our Sweet Potatoes with Red Lentils and Coconut (page 159).

GRAINS, NUTS, AND SEEDS

Amaranth is similar to quinoa in that it is a gluten-free seed (often used like a grain) as well as a complete protein. 1 cup of amaranth contains 5 grams of fiber and approximately 251 calories. It is a good source of B vitamins, calcium, iron, and zinc. Try our Simple Amaranth Porridge (page 32) for an easy breakfast.

Buckwheat groats are similar to grains but are actually kernels that have a lot of protein and are gluten free. Unlike raw buckwheat groats that are edible after an overnight soak, toasted buckwheat groats, also known as kasha, must be boiled and cooked. Raw buckwheat groats get blended into a creamy slurry in our Raw Blended Buckwheat and Chia Porridge with Raspberries, Apples, and Kiwi (page 33).

Chia seeds are used as a thickener in many recipes, but they are quite nutritious! Unlike flaxseeds, which must be ground to reap the most benefits, chia seeds can be absorbed by the body when consumed as a whole seed or ground. Chia seeds contain 11 grams of protein per 2 tablespoons. If you have difficulty swallowing, be sure to consume chia seeds only after they have been soaking in a liquid. See chia seeds featured in our Vanilla Almond Chia Seed Shake (page 175).

Farro falls somewhere between rice and pasta. Although it is not a complete protein like quinoa, farro has more protein than brown rice and has a nice nutty flavor. See this grain featured in our Very Veggie Farro Salad (page 69).

Flax meal is produced from ground flaxseeds, allowing more complete and easier absorption than consuming the full seed. Flax contains fiber, omega-3 fatty acids, and lignans, which may have protective effects against breast, prostate, and colon cancer. If you cannot find flax meal at the grocery, you can make your own flax meal in a coffee grinder and store it in a closed container. Flaxseeds are found in our Berry Banana Nut Butter Bowl (page 34) and in the crust of the Mini Ricotta Coconut Fruit Pies with Hazelnut Crust (page 200).

Quinoa is a quick-cooking (cooks in 15 minutes!) gluten-free seed. It is a nutritionally dense complete protein, which means that it has all nine essential amino acids. Check out our favorites, the Eggy Quinoa Patties (page 53) and the Quinoa Bowl with Sliced Avocado and Yogurt Dressing (page 68).

Seeds and seed butters, such as pumpkin, sunflower, sesame, and poppy, are a wonderful addition to the diet, as they provide healthy fats, fiber, and protein. Add seeds to salads, pastas, smoothies, and oatmeal for a bite of texture. Or try spreading tahini (sesame paste) or sunflower seed butter on toast, mixing into dips, or swirling into oatmeal, smoothies, and baked goods for a creamy twist. We mix tahini into our Avocado Mango Smoothie (page 170), and we like to sprinkle toasted sesame seeds over the Thai-Style Vegetable Strand Salad (page 71).

MEAT ALTERNATIVES AND FLAVORINGS

Nutritional yeast is great way to create a cheesy flavor in vegan recipes. It has 6 grams of protein in 2 tablespoons and is a great source of vitamin B_{12} and folic acid. Sprinkle some over popcorn, over buttered toast, on top of spaghetti, in soups or sauces, or on top of pizza. Since it is a version of yeast, be sure to approve with your physician and registered dietitian before using if you have a low white blood cell count and are immune compromised (also called neutropenic) or have not used before. Find nutritional yeast in our Vegan Mushroom Breakfast Burritos (page 63).

Tempeh is a fermented soy product with a strong, savory, nutty flavor. Unlike tofu, tempeh is firm, making it good on the grill. Because of its nutty flavor, try marinating it in soy sauce, ginger, or vinegar and cooking it by baking or panfrying until crispy. Try our Tempeh Kebabs with Homemade Barbecue Sauce (page 134).

Tofu is made from soybeans and is rich in iron, calcium, and protein. Tofu is sold in a variety of consistencies that range from silken to super or extra-firm. With its mild flavor and range in consistency, tofu absorbs the taste of whatever you cook it in and can be used in sauces, desserts, and entrées. Whip up a quick Tofu Ricotta (page 225), to use as a filling in lasagna, crumble tofu into a pan and make our Tofu Scramble with Pesto and Roasted Cherry Tomatoes (page 60), or make a simple Baked Tofu and Broccoli over Wild Rice (page 136).

Seitan is a textured wheat protein that is often a main player in "fake meat" products. While this is an excellent option if you are trying to cut down on soy consumption, seitan is made from wheat gluten and it cannot be used if you are on a gluten-free diet. The Seitan, Apple, and Broccoli Breakfast Hash (page 62) and the Seitan Teriyaki Lettuce Wraps (page 133) will turn anyone into a seitan lover in no time.

Nutritional Comparison of Proteins

The following chart compares the calories, fat, and protein content in both plant- and animal-based protein sources. Use this as a guide to gauge nutritional content when swapping in various protein sources in recipes.

	Calories	Grams of Fat	Grams of Protein
Tofu—4 oz (½ cup)	75	4–7	7
Seitan—4 oz (½ cup)	170	2	25
Tempeh—4 oz (½ cup)	160	9	15
Beans—4 oz (½ cup)	125	0–4	7–10
Lentils—4 oz (½ cup)	115	0–3	7
Turkey—3 oz	135–225	3–21	21
Chicken—3 oz	135–225	3–21	21
Shrimp—3 oz	135	3–9	21
Fish—3 oz	135	3–9	21
Beef—3 oz	135–225	3–21	21

Milk and Milk Alternatives

Throughout the cookbook, whenever a recipe calls for milk, we tend not to put the type of milk. We want to encourage you to use the type of milk that most fits your nutritional needs and specific tastes. The following chart compares some of the popular types of milks on the market. Please read the descriptions below the chart to learn more about the different components and properties of each type.

Whole Milk: Whole milk contains the full amount of fat and calories and has the boldest flavor and creamiest texture of the milks. Use whole milk if you are trying to gain weight.

Reduced-/Low-fat Milk: Reduced-fat milk contains 2% milk fat, whereas low-fat milk contains 1% milk fat. These milks are creamier than skim milk and are lower in calories than whole milk.

	Calories per cup	Grams Fat per cup	Grams Protein per cup	Milligrams Calcium per cup
Whole milk and Lactose Free Whole Milk	150	8	8	276
Reduced Fat 2% Milk and Lactose Free Reduced Fat Milk	120	5	8	300
Low Fat 1% Milk and Lactose Free Low Fat Milk	100	2	8	300
Skim Milk and Lactose Free Skim Milk	80	0	8	300
Soy Milk	130	4	8	350 (fortified)
Almond Milk	40	3	1	200 (fortified)
Cashew Milk	25	2	1	450 (fortified)
Coconut Milk	45	4.5	0	500 (fortified)
Hemp Milk	140	5	3	500 (fortified)
Rice Milk	120	2	1	20 or 300 (fortified)

Skim Milk: Also called nonfat or fat-free milk, this milk is light in taste and low in calories.

Lactose-free Milk: This milk still contains dairy but an enzyme called lactase has been added to help break down the lactose in milk (lactose is what can give people gastrointestinal irritation, such as gas, bloating, and diarrhea). There are other nondairy alternatives to lactose-free milk below if you are lactose intolerant or dairy free.

Soy Milk: Soy milk is the thickest of the nondairy milks and can have a sweet taste. It also contains the highest amount of protein of the nondairy milks. Flavors vary and can include unsweetened, original, vanilla, and chocolate.

Almond Milk: Almond milk is a bit milder in taste compared to other milks. It contains more calcium than dairy milk, and while it contains vitamins D and E, an 8-ounce glass of almond milk only has about 1 gram of protein.

Cashew Milk: Cashew milk is a great alternative to almond milk. It is creamy but still low calorie. Cashew milk tends to be fortified with calcium, but it is low in protein. Take cashew milk to the next level and try our recipe for Cashew Cream (page 222).

Coconut Milk: This milk has the same creamy texture as whole milk but it is higher in saturated fat—about 4 grams in 1 cup—than other milks. At the store, you can find coconut milk beverages in the dairy aisle; canned coconut milk, which has a thicker consistency and is often used in curries and baking, is found in either the Asian or baking section.

Hemp Milk: Hemp milk is made out of hemp seeds, which are high in omega-3 fatty acids. Shake the container well before using to avoid any thick or grainy bits in the milk. If you love the taste of hemp milk, you can find hemp seeds, sometimes called hemp hearts, at the store. Sprinkle them over your favorite foods just as you would chia seeds.

Rice Milk: Made from boiled rice, rice milk is dairy free and safe for those who suffer from lactose intolerance. Rice milk has more carbohydrates than cow's milk and is also lower in calcium and protein. Plan to add more of these nutrients to your meals with other ingredients.

Oils

When perusing your pantry for which oil to cook with, it is important to know the differences between various oils. Start with the heart healthy extra-virgin olive oil, a staple of the Mediterranean diet, as your go-to oil.

Extra-virgin Olive Oil: Extra-virgin olive oil is a fruity-flavored oil that is good for making dressings and dips, and is safe to cook over medium heat.

Canola Oil: A mild-flavored oil that is great for high-heat cooking and frying. Canola oil is a good source of alpha linolenic acid (ALA), a type of omega-3 fatty acid, which is a heart-healthy fat.

Coconut Oil: Great for high-heat cooking and dairy-free baking. Note the saturated fat content in coconut oil is higher than in other vegetables oils, so use in moderation. This oil is helpful for those with trouble digesting fats, because it contains medium-chain triglycerides which are more readily absorbed by the body.

Grapeseed and Safflower Oils: These are great all-purpose oils for high-heat stir-frying and sautéing. They are good sources of polyunsaturated fats and vitamin E. Safflower oil tastes delicious with popcorn!

Peanut Oil: A slightly nutty yet mild oil with a medium-high smoke point. Can be used in stir-frying or baking.

Dairy-free Butter or Margarine: For those looking for a more traditional take on lactose-free butter, try using a dairy-free margarine. Great for baking and spreading on toast. Be sure to look for margarines that do not have any trans fat because of artery-clogging properties.

Sweeteners and Spices

Dates can be used as a natural form of sweetener, as their juicy skin lends a caramel-like flavor. Dates also contain fiber and potassium. Pop a few dates when you feel a sweet craving, split some dates and spoon almond butter in the center for a nutrient-dense snack, or chop them up and add to your favorite baked goods. We use dates in our Sweet Banana Date Oat Shake (page 172) and our Carrot, Date, and Chickpea Salad (page 72).

Maple Syrup can be substituted for sugar in most recipes. Be sure to use pure maple syrup, not "pancake syrup." It contains more minerals than table sugar and also has small amounts of polyphenols, which are antioxidants that help reduce inflammation. Try it in baked goods or drizzled into oatmeal or our Maple Berry Breakfast Parfait (page 35).

Honey is a sweetener that can be used in baked goods, sauces, smoothies, and other beverages. Honey has a distinct flavor and viscous texture, and it can be soothing to mouth sores. Try it in the Simple Amaranth Porridge (page 32), the Juicy Grilled Summer Peaches (page 210), or the Cinnamon Honey Baked Bananas (page 197).

Agave Nectar can dissolve easily in liquids, making it a great sweetening option for smoothies and drinks. Try it in a homemade peanut sauce or sweet marinade, too.

Molasses is a deeply colored sugar syrup traditionally seen in gingerbread, cookies, and barbecue sauces. Some people like to drizzle it into oatmeal or yogurt, but a little goes a long way with this strong sweetener. Blackstrap molasses is an even darker, slightly more bitter syrup that is often used to help people meet their iron and calcium needs. Try our favorite recipes featuring molasses, such as our Multi-Bran Sour Cream Muffins (page 44) and our Tempeh Kebabs with Homemade Barbecue Sauce (page 134).

Salt may not technically be classified as a spice, but the type of salt you use when cooking is important. In our recipes, we do not explicitly list the type of salt to use because we want you to choose what works for you. We recommend a fine sea salt or kosher salt for your everyday go-to salt needs. Larger crystals of sea salt are great for sprinkling over a finished dish. If you want to go gourmet, try experimenting with flavored salts, such as smoked salt or pink salt.

Cardamom is a very strong spice, so you only need to add a very small amount to recipes to start tasting it. The flavor can lend a sweet spiciness, reminiscent of chai to baked goods, beverages, and savory foods. Use it in our Peach Cardamom Honeyed Yogurt (page 36) or our Hint of Cardamom Spinach Gratin (page 184).

Turmeric is an earthy spice that gives a warm yellow color to such dishes as rice, lentils, soups, and curries. A pinch of turmeric can also be added to beverages, such as milk, smoothies, and tea. It's also a terrific addition to the oil used to cook eggs or French toast, for a little extra flavor. Researchers are currently studying a component of turmeric known as curcumin, which is thought to possess anti-inflammatory properties. Find turmeric in our Hearty Tomato Lentil Soup (page 153) and our Asparagus Potato Curry (page 157).

Saffron is a special spice that looks like little red threads. The taste can be described as a grassy or haylike honey. Saffron can be quite expensive; however; you need only a small amount to make a recipe shine. Try it in our Veggie Paella (page 97).

Essential Kitchen Equipment and Cookware

It is important to have an arsenal of basic kitchen equipment and cookware to help make recipe preparation easier and more efficient. Following are some of our favorite tools that keep us cooking, day in and day out.

Kitchen Scissors: For snipping herbs or trimming fat from chicken.

Collapsible Vegetable Steamer Basket: Inexpensive and fits in a medium-size saucepan.

Colander: For draining pasta and rinsing vegetables, beans, and certain grains.

Spiralizer or Julienne Peeler: A great way to make vegetable pastas or to add fun vegetable strands to salads.

Cutting Boards: Try to have at least two separate cutting boards—one for meat, one for vegetables and other nonmeat products. Having a plastic board will allow you to sanitize them regularly in the dishwasher.

Glass: All glass is inert, nontoxic, and safe. Glass is the perfect material for storing leftovers or snacks.

Stainless Steel: Safe, nonreactive, and affordable, stainless steel is a great material to use for cookware.

Cast Iron: Cast iron has been the go-to material cookware for generations. It is durable, simple in build, and has even heating and good heat retention.

Cast iron tends to rust, so it needs to be "seasoned" with oil before it is used. To clean the skillet, wipe it down with a cloth or nylon dish brush. You can run it under water, but try not to use soap, as soap will undo the "season" on the pan. Wipe the skillet dry with a paper towel or rag, and lightly coat with oil.

Parchment Paper: This all-purpose paper is an easy nonstick liner for baking. Cooking in parchment paper is a great way to prepare healthy and flavorful foods, especially fish and vegetables. Wrapping a piece of fish in the paper lets the fish steam, allowing it to retain more nutrients than baking, frying, or cooking on a skillet.

Part 2
Let's Cook!
Recipes

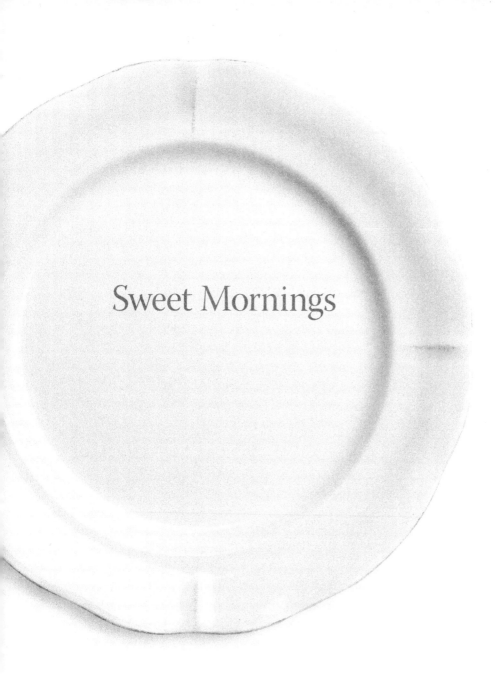

Sweet Mornings

Apple Crumble Baked Oatmeal

Time: Prep: 15 minutes; Cook: 40–45 minutes
Serves 6

Oatmeal is a great and soothing breakfast for anyone experiencing digestive issues; this version is easy and delicious, and extra comforting with its warm apple and spice flavors. Leftover baked oatmeal can be reheated the following day and served in a bowl with a little milk, yogurt, or nut butter.

Unsalted butter or oil, for baking dish

2 cups rolled oats

1 teaspoon baking powder

½ tablespoon ground cinnamon

¼ teaspoon ground nutmeg

½ teaspoon salt

2 cups milk

¼ cup pure maple syrup

1 large egg

2 tablespoons unsalted butter or coconut oil, melted

2 teaspoons vanilla extract

3 apples, peeled, cored, and cut in half

For the crumble topping

½ cup roughly chopped walnuts or other nut

1 tablespoon unsalted butter or coconut oil, melted

Pinch of salt

1 tablespoon light or dark brown sugar

1. Preheat the oven to 375°F and grease a 9 by 9-inch baking dish with unsalted butter or oil.
2. Place the oats, baking powder, cinnamon, nutmeg, and salt in a bowl and stir together. Pour this mixture into the prepared baking dish.
3. In another bowl, combine the milk, maple syrup, egg, melted butter, and vanilla. Whisk together completely. Slowly pour this over the oats.
4. Tuck the apple halves into the oats, cut side down.
5. Combine the crumble ingredients in a small bowl, then sprinkle over the top of the oats and apples.
6. Bake for 40 to 45 minutes, or until the center is cooked through and the crumble is deep golden and caramelized. Let cool slightly, then serve with extra maple syrup, brown sugar, milk, or yogurt.

Nutritional Analysis: Calories 347, Total Fat 16 g, Saturated Fat 5 g, Cholesterol 55 mg, Sodium 301 mg, Carbohydrates 45 g, Dietary Fiber 5 g, Protein 9 g

Lack of Appetite	+
Nausea, Vomiting, or Heartburn	+
Constipation	+
Diarrhea	+
Fatigue	+
Mouth Sores	+
Dry Mouth	+
Chewing or Swallowing Difficulty	+
Taste Aversion—Sweet	
Taste Aversion—Sour & Bitter	
Lack of Taste	+
Smells Bother	+

Sweet Baked Banana Oatmeal

Time: Prep: 15 minutes; Cook: 40–45 minutes
Serves 4

This sweet morning treat is inspired by our love of dessert and also works as a dessert when topped with frozen yogurt or ice cream. With soluble fiber from the oats and bananas, and potassium from the bananas, the recipe is great for combating diarrhea. Store leftover oatmeal in the refrigerator for up to 3 days and reheat it in the microwave or oven.

Unsalted butter or oil, for baking dish	1¼ cups milk
¾ cup rolled oats	1 tablespoon canola oil
¼ cup oat flour	1 tablespoon pure maple syrup
1 teaspoon ground cinnamon, plus more for banana topping	(or other sweetener)
	3 small, firm, ripe bananas,
½ teaspoon baking powder	chopped
½ cup chopped walnut halves (optional)	1 teaspoon vanilla extract

1. Preheat the oven to 350°F and lightly grease a 9 by 9-inch baking dish with unsalted butter or oil.
2. Stir the oats, oat flour, cinnamon, baking powder, walnuts (if using), and milk in a large bowl until combined. Transfer to the prepared baking dish and set aside.
3. Prepare the bananas: Heat a skillet over medium-high heat and place the oil and maple syrup in the skillet. When the mixture starts to simmer and bubble, add the chopped bananas and stir well until coated in syrup. Sprinkle with a few pinches of cinnamon. Sauté for about 5 minutes, lowering the heat if necessary, until the bananas soften. Remove from the heat and stir in the vanilla.
4. Spoon the banana mixture over the oatmeal mixture.
5. Bake, uncovered, for 40 to 45 minutes, or until the top is golden. After cooling slightly, slice the oatmeal into squares or spoon it into bowls.

Nutritional Analysis: Calories 320, Total Fat 16 g, Saturated Fat 2 g, Cholesterol 4 mg, Sodium 104 mg, Carbohydrates 41 g, Dietary Fiber 5 g, Protein 8 g

Sidebar (left margin):
+ Lack of Appetite
+ Nausea, Vomiting, or Heartburn
+ Constipation
+ Diarrhea
+ Fatigue
+ Mouth Sores
+ Dry Mouth
+ Chewing or Swallowing Difficulty
  Taste Aversion—Sweet
+ Taste Aversion—Sour & Bitter
+ Lack of Taste
+ Smells Bother

AB & B Oats ◑

Time: Prep: 15 minutes; Cook: 5 minutes
Serves 1

"AB & B" stands for Almond Butter & Banana, a delicious and healthful combination. Substitute any favorite nut butter for the almond butter. Mashing the banana and mixing it into the oats adds volume and creaminess. Leftovers keep in the refrigerator for 3 days. Reheat in the microwave, or enjoy cold, adding an extra splash of milk as needed.

½ cup rolled oats	1 teaspoon packed light or dark brown
¾ to 1 cup water or milk	sugar or pure maple syrup
Pinch of salt	Pinch of ground cinnamon
1 small banana	½ tablespoon almond butter

1. Combine the oats, water, and salt in a microwave-safe bowl (for microwave preparation) or a small saucepan (for stovetop).
2. Microwave the oats on high power for 2 to 3 minutes, stopping to stir the oats halfway through. Alternatively, boil them over medium heat on the stovetop for 2 minutes. Check the consistency and continue to heat over low heat, stirring often, until the oats are fluffy and thick, for another 2 to 3 minutes.
3. In a small bowl, mash the banana and add to the oats. Heat for another 30 seconds in the microwave or on the stovetop.
4. Stir in the brown sugar and cinnamon. Top with the almond butter.

Nutritional Analysis (prepared using water): Calories 306, Total Fat 8 g, Saturated Fat 1 g, Cholesterol 0 mg, Sodium 56 mg, Carbohydrates 56 g, Dietary Fiber 7 g, Protein 8 g

Lack of Appetite	+
Nausea, Vomiting, or Heartburn	+
Constipation	+
Diarrhea	+
Fatigue	+
Mouth Sores	+
Dry Mouth	+
Chewing or Swallowing Difficulty	+
Taste Aversion— Sweet	
Taste Aversion— Sour & Bitter	
Lack of Taste	+
Smells Bother	+

Simple Amaranth Porridge ①

Time: Prep: 5 minutes; Cook: 20–25 minutes
Serves 4

Amaranth is a seed that contains protein and calcium, and it cooks up into a delicious porridge. Serve with fresh or dried fruit, lavender-flavored or regular honey, and ground cinnamon. Honey is especially soothing for mouth sores.

....

1 cup amaranth seeds	regular honey
4 cups water or milk (or a mix of both)	Fresh or dried fruit
1 to 2 tablespoons lavender-flavored or	Pinch of ground cinnamon

1. Combine the amaranth seeds and water in a saucepan. Bring to a boil over medium heat, then lower the heat to a simmer and cook, stirring, until creamy, for 20 to 25 minutes. Stir constantly during the last 5 minutes of cooking (the porridge will sputter).
2. If the porridge seems thick, add more water or milk. Stir in the honey, fruit, and cinnamon before serving. Add an extra splash of milk to each bowl, as desired.

Nutritional Analysis (as prepared with 2 cups water and 2 cups 1% low-fat milk, not including fruit): Calories 254, Total Fat 5 g, Saturated Fat 1 g, Cholesterol 6 mg, Sodium 61 mg, Carbohydrates 44 g, Dietary Fiber 3 g, Protein 11 g

Stretch and Save: Use leftover porridge to make tasty amaranth cookies. Combine 2 cups of leftover amaranth porridge, 1 cup of all-purpose flour, ½ cup of melted butter, 3 to 4 tablespoons of honey or pure maple syrup, a pinch of salt, 1 teaspoon of vanilla extract, and 1 beaten large egg. Portion the dough into small mounds on a parchment-lined baking sheet. Bake for 12 to 15 minutes in a preheated 350°F oven, or until just starting to brown. Remove from the oven and let cool. Store any remaining cookies in the refrigerator.

Nutritionist's Favorite to Savor
This recipe is my breakfast favorite because it uses an uncommon seed, amaranth, to cook up a surprisingly delicious high-protein porridge. With just a few ingredients, this recipe is approachable and can accommodate a variety of nutrition-related symptoms commonly experienced by cancer patients. Prepare a batch on one morning and enjoy throughout the week.

Side margin labels

- Lack of Appetite +
- Nausea, Vomiting, or Heartburn +
- Constipation +
- Diarrhea +
- Fatigue +
- Mouth Sores +
- Dry Mouth +
- Chewing or Swallowing Difficulty +
- Taste Aversion— Sweet
- Taste Aversion— Sour & Bitter
- Lack of Taste
- Smells Bother +

Raw Blended Buckwheat and Chia Porridge with Raspberries, Apples, and Kiwi ⓘ

Time: Prep: 15 minutes + an overnight soak
Serves 4

This no-cook porridge is an easy-to-make breakfast that just requires a little preparation the night before. If sensitive to spices, reduce or omit the cardamom, cinnamon, or nutmeg. This porridge will keep in the refrigerator for up to 5 days. Portion into individual jars for easy access.

For the porridge
1 cup raw buckwheat groats
⅓ cup almond meal or
    ground almonds
¼ cup chia seeds
2 apples, peeled, cored, and chopped
½ cup fresh or frozen raspberries
⅛ teaspoon ground cardamom
¼ teaspoon ground cinnamon

Pinch of ground nutmeg
1 tablespoon pure maple syrup

Toppings
2 tablespoons chopped or slivered
    almonds
2 kiwis, peeled and chopped
Drizzle of pure maple syrup or honey
    (optional)

1. Soak the buckwheat overnight in 2 to 3 cups of water.
2. The next day, drain and rinse the buckwheat. It may look a little slimy, but that is normal.
3. Place the buckwheat along with the almond meal, chia seeds, apples, raspberries, cardamom, cinnamon, nutmeg, and maple syrup in a high-speed blender and blend until it becomes creamy and smooth in texture. Add up to 1 cup more of water, if needed, a little bit at a time, until the desired consistency is reached.
4. Scoop into jars or bowls and add the toppings.

Nutritional Analysis: Calories 352, Total Fat 11 g, Saturated Fat 1 g, Cholesterol 0 mg, Sodium 14 mg, Carbohydrates 59 g, Dietary Fiber 11 g, Protein 10 g

Lack of Appetite	+
Nausea, Vomiting, or Heartburn	
Constipation	+
Diarrhea	
Fatigue	+
Mouth Sores	+
Dry Mouth	+
Chewing or Swallowing Difficulty	+
Taste Aversion— Sweet	
Taste Aversion— Sour & Bitter	
Lack of Taste	+
Smells Bother	+

Berry Banana Nut Butter Bowl ◐

Time: 10 minutes
Serves 2

This flavorful breakfast bowl is quick to prepare and delicious to eat; high-fiber berries and ground flaxseeds help with digestion. Use thawed frozen berries when fresh berries are not in season. Don't have any peanut butter? Use almond butter, sunflower seed butter, or yogurt instead.

½ cup sliced strawberries	½ cup sliced bananas
½ cup blueberries	2 tablespoons peanut butter
½ cup raspberries	1 tablespoon ground flaxseeds

1. Divide the berries and bananas equally between two bowls.
2. Dollop each bowl with 1 tablespoon of peanut butter, sprinkle each with ½ tablespoon of flaxseeds, and enjoy.

Nutritional Analysis: Calories 195, Total Fat 10 g, Saturated Fat 2 g, Cholesterol 0 mg, Sodium 76 mg, Carbohydrates 25 g, Dietary Fiber 7 g, Protein 6 g

Lack of Appetite +

Nausea, Vomiting, or Heartburn +

Constipation +

Diarrhea

Fatigue +

Mouth Sores

Dry Mouth +

Chewing or Swallowing Difficulty +

Taste Aversion—Sweet

Taste Aversion—Sour & Bitter

Lack of Taste +

Smells Bother +

Maple Berry Breakfast Parfait ◖

Time: 5 minutes
Serves 2

Feeling fatigued? Here is an easy recipe to make and keep portioned in the fridge for an easy-to-grab meal or snack. For added calories, use whole milk Greek yogurt and extra nuts. This recipe can also work as a healthy dessert. For a sweeter touch, try topping with a drizzle of honey or a scoop of whipped cream. Parfaits will keep for up to 5 days in the refrigerator.

2 cups low-fat plain Greek yogurt	1 cup raspberries, strawberries, or blueberries
1 tablespoon pure maple syrup	⅔ cup granola
½ teaspoon vanilla extract	2 tablespoons sliced almonds

1. Mix the Greek yogurt with the maple syrup and vanilla.
2. Using four small jars, start with a layer of yogurt, then berries, then granola and almonds. Repeat the layers once more, or until the jars are full. Sprinkle any leftover almonds and granola on the top and serve. Alternatively, divide the yogurt between two bowls and top with berries, granola, and sliced almonds.

Nutritional Analysis: Calories 446, Total Fat 18 g, Saturated Fat 5 g, Cholesterol 15 mg, Sodium 87 mg, Carbohydrates 46 g, Dietary Fiber 8 g, Protein 27 g

Symptom	
Lack of Appetite	+
Nausea, Vomiting, or Heartburn	+
Constipation	+
Diarrhea	
Fatigue	+
Mouth Sores	
Dry Mouth	+
Chewing or Swallowing Difficulty	+
Taste Aversion—Sweet	
Taste Aversion—Sour & Bitter	+
Lack of Taste	+
Smells Bother	+

Peach Cardamom Honeyed Yogurt ①

Time: 5 minutes
Serves 2

Use peaches canned in fruit juice, for added tenderness. For an extra-frosty breakfast or snack, place these ingredients and a few ice cubes in a blender and enjoy as a smoothie.

....

1½ cups or 2 (6-ounce) containers
   low-fat plain Greek yogurt
1 to 2 tablespoons honey, plus more
   for drizzling (optional)

¼ teaspoon ground ginger
⅛ teaspoon ground cardamom
2 fresh peaches, pitted and sliced

....

1. In a medium-size bowl, combine the yogurt, honey, ginger, and cardamom. Stir until smooth.
2. Divide the peach slices equally between two bowls or jars. Spoon the yogurt into the bowls and drizzle each bowl with a little extra honey, if desired.

Nutritional Analysis: Calories 221, Total Fat 4 g, Saturated Fat 2 g, Cholesterol 11 mg, Sodium 57 mg, Carbohydrates 34 g, Dietary Fiber 2 g, Protein 16 g

---

Sidebar (left margin):

+ Lack of Appetite

+ Nausea, Vomiting, or Heartburn

+ Constipation

Diarrhea

+ Fatigue

Mouth Sores

+ Dry Mouth

+ Chewing or Swallowing Difficulty

Taste Aversion—Sweet

Taste Aversion—Sour & Bitter

+ Lack of Taste

+ Smells Bother

Pineapple and Papaya "Brûlée" ◐

Time: Prep: 10 minutes; Cook: 5 minutes
Serves 4

Papaya and pineapple contain enzymes that are helpful for digestion—papain and bromelain, respectively. To save time on preparation, look for precut fruit in the produce section of your grocery store, but know they can be pricier than buying the whole fruit.

½ cup chopped ripe papaya	1 cup low-fat vanilla yogurt
½ cup chopped pineapple	2 tablespoons light or dark brown sugar
Grated zest of 2 limes	1 tablespoon freshly squeezed lime juice

1. Set the broiler to HIGH. Get out a baking sheet.
2. Cut the fruit into bite-size pieces. Place in a bowl and stir in the lime zest, then divide the cut fruit among four small ramekins.
3. Top with the yogurt, ¼ cup per ramekin, smoothing out the top as you go. Add a little more, if needed, to get a smooth top.
4. Crumble a thin layer of brown sugar over each, about ½ tablespoon per ramekin. Drizzle ½ teaspoon of lime juice over each.
5. Place the ramekins on the baking sheet and broil for 2 to 3 minutes, or just until the topping melts and browns. Remove from the broiler and let cool slightly. Serve.

Nutritional Analysis: Calories 80, Total Fat 1 g, Saturated Fat 1 g, Cholesterol 4 mg, Sodium 44 mg, Carbohydrates 16 g, Dietary Fiber 1 g, Protein 3 g

Lack of Appetite +

Nausea, Vomiting, or Heartburn

Constipation +

Diarrhea

Fatigue +

Mouth Sores

Dry Mouth

Chewing or Swallowing Difficulty +

Taste Aversion— Sweet +

Taste Aversion— Sour & Bitter

Lack of Taste +

Smells Bother +

Quinoa Coconut Pancakes ◑

Time: Prep: 10 minutes; Cook: 15 minutes
Serves 4 (makes 12 small pancakes or 8 medium)

Quinoa flour adds extra protein and fiber to these pancakes (and it makes them gluten free [note: if you use whole wheat flour, they will not be gluten free]), but fear not, the pancakes are still just as fluffy as a traditional pancake. Use coconut milk in the recipe, for extra coconut flavor. For extra texture, top with rolled oats while cooking. Store leftover pancakes in the refrigerator for up to 2 days or in the freezer, individually wrapped, for up to 1 month. Pop one or two in a toaster oven or microwave for breakfast.

1½ cups quinoa flour or
    whole wheat flour
½ cup coconut flour
4 teaspoons baking powder
½ teaspoon salt
2 tablespoons sugar
3 tablespoons canola oil, mashed
    banana, or applesauce

1 teaspoon vanilla extract
2½ cups milk
4 teaspoons canola oil or nonstick
    cooking spray, to cook the pancakes
¼ cup shredded coconut
Pure maple syrup, jam, or fresh fruit,
    for serving

1. In a small bowl, whisk together the quinoa flour, coconut flour, baking powder, salt, and sugar.
2. In another small bowl, whisk together the canola oil, vanilla, and milk.
3. Pour the wet ingredients into the dry and stir to combine.
4. Heat a skillet over medium heat and place 1 teaspoon of canola oil in the skillet, or spray with cooking spray.
5. Pour the batter into the pan to make three small or two medium-size pancakes. Sprinkle 1 teaspoon of shredded coconut on top of each pancake.
6. When bubbles form and the edges start to cook, flip and cook for about 30 seconds more.
7. Transfer the cooked pancakes to an ovenproof plate or baking sheet and place in a warm (about 150°F) oven until the remaining pancakes are cooked and ready to serve.
8. Serve the pancakes drizzled with maple syrup or with jam and fresh fruit. Greek yogurt and nut butters also make great toppings.

Lack of
Appetite

Nausea,
Vomiting, or
Heartburn

Constipation

Diarrhea

Fatigue

Mouth
Sores

Dry
Mouth

Chewing or
Swallowing
Difficulty

Taste
Aversion—
Sweet

Taste
Aversion—
Sour & Bitter

Lack of
Taste

Smells
Bother

Nutritional Analysis: Calories 86, Total Fat 6.7 g, Saturated Fat 1.5 g, Cholesterol 4 mg, Sodium 123 mg, Carbohydrates 5.6 g, Dietary Fiber 2 g, Protein 1.7 g

Apple Butternut Squash Yogurt Pancakes ①

Time: Prep: 15 minutes; Cook: 10 minutes
Serves 3 (makes 12 small pancakes or 6 large)

+	Lack of Appetite
+	Nausea, Vomiting, or Heartburn
+	Constipation
+	Diarrhea
+	Fatigue
+	Mouth Sores
+	Dry Mouth
+	Chewing or Swallowing Difficulty
+	Taste Aversion— Sweet
	Taste Aversion— Sour & Bitter
+	Lack of Taste
+	Smells Bother

These not-too-sweet pancakes bring warmth to cool fall mornings for you and your family. They are also a great option for a light dinner meal. Orange-fleshed winter squashes are rich in beta-carotene that your body converts to vitamin A and uses as an antioxidant.

1 small butternut or acorn squash
1 large apple
⅓ cup plain yogurt
1 large egg
¼ cup milk
1 cup all-purpose or whole wheat flour
1 teaspoon baking powder
1 teaspoon baking soda
1 teaspoon ground cinnamon
3 teaspoons canola oil or
    nonstick cooking spray,
    to cook the pancakes

1. Cut the ends off the squash, then peel. Next, cut it in half and scoop out the seeds. Grate the squash, using a cheese grater or food processor, until you have about 3 cups' worth. Place the grated squash in a microwave-safe bowl, add 2 tablespoons of water, and cover with a plate. Steam in the microwave on high power for 3 minutes to soften, adding more water, if needed. Drain any extra water and let cool slightly. Transfer to a large bowl.
2. Core and grate the apple and add to the squash mixture.
3. In a separate bowl, stir together the yogurt, egg, and milk and then add to the squash mixture.
4. In a separate bowl, sift together the flour, baking powder, baking soda, and cinnamon. Add to the squash mixture and stir until combined.
5. Heat a pan over medium heat and place 1 teaspoon of canola oil in the pan or spray with cooking spray. Using a ladle or a spoon, drop the batter onto the pan into pancake rounds. Flip when the bottom is golden brown (usually when bubbles form and the edges start to cook) and cook until the other side is golden.
6. Transfer the cooked pancakes to an ovenproof plate or baking sheet and place in a warm oven (about 150°F) until the remaining pancakes are cooked and ready to serve.

Nutritional Analysis: Calories 368, Total Fat 8 g, Saturated Fat 1 g, Cholesterol 74 mg, Sodium 662 mg, Carbohydrates 68 g, Dietary Fiber 10 g, Protein 10 g

Nutritionist's Favorite to Savor
This recipe is my favorite because pancakes always feel festive. Since the recipe calls for both grated apple and winter squash, it is a great way to get some fruits and vegetables into the morning meal. Aim to include at least one fruit and/or vegetable with each meal and snack to optimize your plant-based intake.

Eggless Banana Battered French Toast ①

Time: Prep: 10 minutes; Cook: 10 minutes
Serves 3

+	Lack of Appetite
+	Nausea, Vomiting, or Heartburn
+	Constipation
+	Diarrhea
+	Fatigue
+	Mouth Sores
+	Dry Mouth
+	Chewing or Swallowing Difficulty
+	Taste Aversion— Sweet
+	Taste Aversion— Sour & Bitter
+	Lack of Taste
+	Smells Bother

For additional fiber, use whole wheat bread. Top with chopped nuts, for added protein. To make the recipe vegan, use nondairy milk instead of cow's milk and cook the French toast in oil instead of butter. The batter will keep for 1 day in the refrigerator.

....

1 ripe banana, mashed
½ cup milk
1 tablespoon canola or coconut oil, or unsalted butter

6 slices bread (any kind)
Handful of blueberries or raspberries
Pure maple syrup

....

1. Blend the bananas and milk in a blender or whisk together vigorously by hand. Pour into a large bowl.
2. Place a nonstick skillet over medium heat and heat the oil.
3. One at a time, dip the slices of bread in the banana mixture and let them soak on both sides.
4. Shake off any excess liquid and add the drenched bread to the skillet until browned on both sides. You may need to cook this in batches, depending on the size of your pan.
5. Top with berries and drizzle with a little maple syrup. Tastes delicious with shredded coconut or ground cinnamon sprinkled on top, too!

Nutritional Analysis (does not include toppings): Calories 432, Total Fat 17 g, Saturated Fat 1 g, Cholesterol 83 mg, Sodium 407 mg, Carbohydrates 63 g, Dietary Fiber 2 g, Protein 9 g

Cinnamon Whole Wheat Waffles ⏱

Time: Prep: 10 minutes; Cook: 20 minutes
Serves 6

These waffles can be made ahead, frozen, and reheated whenever a quick, sweet breakfast is needed. Try topping with some peanut butter and chopped bananas for a filling and nutritious start to the day. For a vegan version, use nondairy milk and replace the egg with a flax "egg": Mix 1 tablespoon of ground flaxseeds with 2½ tablespoons of water. Let sit for 5 minutes and use in place of the egg.

1½ cups whole wheat flour	1 teaspoon vanilla extract
2 teaspoons baking powder	1 large egg or 1 flax egg
½ teaspoon baking soda	(see headnote)
½ teaspoon salt	1½ cups milk
1 teaspoon ground cinnamon	⅓ cup canola or vegetable oil
2 tablespoons light or dark brown sugar	Fresh fruit, for topping (optional)

1. Whisk together the flour, baking powder, baking soda, salt, cinnamon, and sugar in a large bowl.
2. In a separate bowl, whisk together the vanilla, egg, milk, and oil.
3. Mix the wet and dry ingredients together, stirring until just combined.
4. Heat a waffle iron according to the manufacturer's instructions and cook the waffles until the batter is all used up. Top with fresh fruit, if using, and enjoy.

Nutritional Analysis: Calories 267, Total Fat 15 g, Saturated Fat 2 g, Cholesterol 39 mg, Sodium 487 mg, Carbohydrates 29 g, Dietary Fiber 3 g, Protein 7 g

Lack of Appetite	+
Nausea, Vomiting, or Heartburn	+
Constipation	+
Diarrhea	+
Fatigue	+
Mouth Sores	+
Dry Mouth	+
Chewing or Swallowing Difficulty	+
Taste Aversion— Sweet	
Taste Aversion— Sour & Bitter	+
Lack of Taste	+
Smells Bother	+

Multi-Bran Sour Cream Muffins

Time: Prep: 15 minutes; Cook: 30 minutes
Makes 16 muffins

Made from the dense outer hull of grains, bran is incredibly rich in protein and fiber, which means it is excellent for digestion. These muffins are great to have on hand as a quick snack to help combat fatigue. Freeze extra muffins in either a resealable plastic bag or an airtight container for up to 1 month.

Unsalted butter or nonstick cooking spray, for muffin tin (optional)	2 large eggs
2 cups wheat bran	⅔ cup milk
1 cup oat bran	⅔ cup low-fat sour cream or plain Greek yogurt
1 cup whole wheat flour	⅓ cup canola oil
2 teaspoons baking soda	⅓ cup molasses
1 teaspoon baking powder	⅓ cup honey
½ teaspoon salt	1 teaspoon vanilla extract

1. Preheat the oven to 375°F. Grease sixteen standard-size muffin cups or line with paper liners.
2. Combine the wheat bran, oat bran, whole wheat flour, baking soda, baking powder, and salt in a large bowl and set aside.
3. In a separate small bowl, combine the eggs, milk, sour cream, canola oil, molasses, honey, and vanilla and mix well.
4. Pour the wet ingredients into the dry and mix with a rubber spatula just until combined.
5. Fill each muffin cup three-quarters full.
6. Bake until a toothpick inserted in the center of a muffin comes out clean, for 20 to 25 minutes. Let the muffins cool in the pan for 10 to 15 minutes, then carefully remove them and serve warm, or let them cool on a wire rack.

Nutritional Analysis: Calories 158, Total Fat 6 g, Saturated Fat 1 g, Cholesterol 28 mg, Sodium 270 mg, Carbohydrates 26 g, Dietary Fiber 5 g, Protein 5 g

Lack of Appetite
Nausea, Vomiting, or Heartburn
Constipation
Diarrhea
Fatigue
Mouth Sores
Dry Mouth
Chewing or Swallowing Difficulty
Taste Aversion—Sweet
Taste Aversion—Sour & Bitter
Lack of Taste
Smells Bother

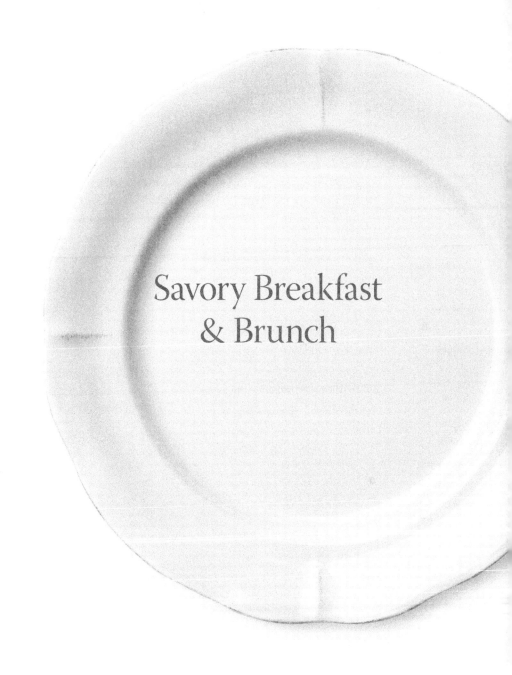

Savory Breakfast
& Brunch

Classic Avocado Toast

Time: 5 minutes
Serves 1

Lack of Appetite	+
Nausea, Vomiting, or Heartburn	+
Constipation	+
Diarrhea	+
Fatigue	+

Avocado is a great source of monounsaturated, heart-healthy fat. For a higher-protein variation, add some cottage cheese on top of the avocado toast. Cooked eggs pair well with avocado toast, too.

1 thick slice of bread

½ ripe avocado, peeled and pitted

Salt

Drizzle of olive oil or lemon juice, or sprinkling of red pepper flakes (optional)

1. Toast the bread.
2. Smash the avocado onto the bread with a fork.
3. Top with salt to taste and any of the optional toppings.

Nutritional Analysis: Calories 269, Total Fat 16 g, Saturated Fat 2 g, Cholesterol 0 mg, Sodium 236 mg, Carbohydrates 26 g, Dietary Fiber 10 g, Protein 7 g

Mouth Sores

Dry Mouth

Chewing or Swallowing Difficulty

Taste Aversion— Sweet

Taste Aversion— Sour & Bitter +

Lack of Taste +

Smells Bother +

Bull's-Eye Skillet Avocado Eggs

Time: Prep: 10 minutes; Cook: 30 minutes
Serves 2

This dish uses avocado halves as an appealing, edible "cup" for eggs. These can also be served as a lighter lunch or dinner meal because of their nutrient density. For someone with a compromised immune system, cook longer, until the yolk is fully cooked.

1 large ripe avocado	1 teaspoon olive oil
2 large eggs	Salt and freshly ground black pepper

1. Cut the avocado in half, remove the pit, and scoop out enough of the flesh to accommodate an entire egg in each hollowed-out peel.
2. Remove a small portion of the outer peel of each avocado half so it sits straight when you set it on a cutting board.
3. Crack and separate the eggs, placing the yolks in two individual ramekins or small cups and both whites together in a small bowl.
4. Heat the olive oil in a lidded skillet over medium-high heat.
5. Add the avocado shells, flesh side down, and sear them, uncovered, for about 30 seconds, or until slightly golden.
6. Flip the avocado shells over and fill the cavities almost to the top with the egg whites.
7. Lower the heat to medium-low, put the lid on, and cook for 15 to 20 minutes, or until the egg whites have turned from clear to white and are almost set.
8. Carefully slide the yolks over the whites and continue cooking for 3 to 5 minutes, or until the yolks are cooked all the way through.
9. Sprinkle with salt and pepper and serve.

Nutritional Analysis: Calories 251, Total Fat 21 g, Saturated Fat 4 g, Cholesterol 215 mg, Sodium 132 mg, Carbohydrates 10 g, Dietary Fiber 7 g, Protein 8 g

Stretch and Save: After you scoop out the flesh to make room for the egg, any leftover avocado can be used to make Classic Avocado Toast (page 46).

Lack of Appetite	+
Nausea, Vomiting, or Heartburn	
Constipation	+
Diarrhea	+
Fatigue	+
Mouth Sores	+
Dry Mouth	+
Chewing or Swallowing Difficulty	+
Taste Aversion—Sweet	
Taste Aversion—Sour & Bitter	+
Lack of Taste	+
Smells Bother	+

Easy-Bake Grab-and-Go Veggie Egg Muffins ⓘ

Time: Prep: 15 minutes; Cook: 15 minutes
Makes 12 muffins

+ Lack of
Appetite

Nausea,
Vomiting, or
Heartburn

+ Constipation

Diarrhea

+ Fatigue

+ Mouth
Sores

+ Dry
Mouth

+ Chewing or
Swallowing
Difficulty

+ Taste
Aversion—
Sweet

Taste
Aversion—
Sour & Bitter

+ Lack of
Taste

+ Smells
Bother

Egg muffins make a great protein-rich snack or a nice addition to eat with a bowl of oatmeal in the morning. This recipe calls for zucchini and spinach, but you can also use whatever vegetables you have on hand. Leftover muffins will keep in the refrigerator for up to 5 days, or wrapped well in the freezer for up to a month. Enjoy leftovers smashed into an English muffin or rolled up in a tortilla with a splash of hot sauce.

Nonstick cooking spray or olive oil,
   for muffin tin
2 teaspoons olive oil
2 scallions, thinly sliced,
   or ¼ small onion, diced
1 medium-size zucchini, finely diced
4 cups roughly chopped spinach leaves

10 large leaves fresh basil,
   cut into thin strips
12 large eggs, beaten
¼ cup grated Pecorino Romano
   or Parmesan cheese
Salt and freshly ground black pepper

1. Preheat the oven to 375°F. Grease twelve standard-size muffin cups with cooking spray or olive oil.
2. Heat the 2 teaspoons of olive oil in a skillet over medium-high heat and lightly sauté the scallion and zucchini for about 5 minutes. Add the spinach and cook until just wilted, for about 2 minutes, then add the basil. Let the vegetables cook for about 5 minutes.
3. In a large bowl, combine the cooked vegetables, beaten eggs, cheese, and a pinch each of salt and pepper. Divide the egg mixture among the prepared muffin cups.
4. Bake for 25 to 30 minutes, or until the eggs are completely cooked. Remove from the oven, wait for 5 minutes, then run a knife or offset spatula around the outside of the muffins and coax them off the bottom.
5. Enjoy warm or place on a wire rack to cool and save for later.

Nutritional Analysis: Calories 182, Total Fat 12 g, Saturated Fat 4 g, Cholesterol 433 mg, Sodium 290 mg, Carbohydrates 5 g, Dietary Fiber 1 g, Protein 14 g

Red and Green Eggs Florentine ⓘ

Time: Prep: 10 minutes; Cook: 10 minutes
Serves 2

Many cancer patients prefer to eat breakfast foods for lunch or dinner over heavier savory options when they have an upset stomach. Try this spin on Eggs Florentine for those times. Soft poached eggs are not recommended for someone with a compromised immune system; substitute a fully cooked boiled or scrambled egg, or poach the egg until the yolk is completely cooked.

1 recipe Yogurt Hollandaise Sauce (page 214)	5 cups fresh baby spinach leaves
1 tablespoon olive oil	Salt and freshly ground black pepper
1 red bell pepper, seeded and sliced	1 tablespoon white, red, or cider vinegar
1 garlic clove, minced	4 large eggs
	2 whole-grain English muffins

1. Make the Yogurt Hollandaise Sauce or prepare it the day before.
2. Heat the olive oil in a skillet over medium heat, add the red pepper slices, and sauté for about 4 minutes, or until tender.
3. Add the garlic and sauté for 30 seconds, until fragrant.
4. Add the spinach in batches and cook down until just wilted. Add salt and black pepper to taste. Set aside.
5. Bring 4 cups of water and vinegar to a boil, then lower the heat to a simmer. This is the egg-poaching liquid. Crack one egg into a small bowl or ramekin. Swirl the water with a spoon to make a vortex and gently pour the egg into it. Cook the egg until the whites are set. Repeat with the remaining eggs.
6. To assemble: Split and toast the English muffins. On a serving plate, top each toasted English muffin half with the sautéed vegetables and a poached egg, then add a spoonful of Yogurt Hollandaise over the top.

Nutritional Analysis (includes 2 tablespoons Yogurt Hollandaise Sauce):
Calories 425, Total Fat 19 g, Saturated Fat 5 g, Cholesterol 501 mg,
Sodium 831 mg, Carbohydrates 43 g, Dietary Fiber 6 g, Protein 22 g

Lack of Appetite	+
Nausea, Vomiting, or Heartburn	
Constipation	+
Diarrhea	
Fatigue	+
Mouth Sores	
Dry Mouth	+
Chewing or Swallowing Difficulty	+
Taste Aversion—Sweet	
Taste Aversion—Sour & Bitter	+
Lack of Taste	+
Smells Bother	+

Roasted Breakfast Potatoes with Tofu Egg Scramble

Time: Prep: 15 minutes; Cook: 30 minutes
Serves 4

Lack of Appetite

Nausea, Vomiting, or Heartburn

Constipation

Diarrhea

Fatigue

Mouth Sores

Dry Mouth

Chewing or Swallowing Difficulty

Taste Aversion— Sweet

Taste Aversion— Sour & Bitter

Lack of Taste

Smells Bother

Replace the tarragon with other herbs of preference, such as parsley, sage, or rosemary. In the mood for some spice? Sprinkle in a few shakes of turmeric, chili powder, or cumin along with the paprika. Leftover potatoes can be saved and served as a side for lunch or dinner. Extra tofu mixture can also be wrapped in a warm tortilla and enjoyed with salsa or a favorite sauce.

1½ pounds potatoes (any variety)
2 tablespoons olive oil
1 teaspoon paprika
1 cup diced soft tofu (not silken tofu)
8 large eggs

1 teaspoon Dijon mustard
1 teaspoon finely chopped
   fresh tarragon
Salt and freshly ground black pepper

1. Preheat the oven to 425°F.
2. Cut the potatoes into ½-inch cubes. Toss with 1 tablespoon of the olive oil and the paprika.
3. Place the potatoes in a single layer on a baking sheet or pan. Bake for 30 minutes, or until roasted and tender.
4. Meanwhile, in a blender, combine the tofu, eggs, mustard, and tarragon. Process until the mixture is smooth.
5. Heat the remaining tablespoon of olive oil in medium-size skillet. Add the egg mixture and cook with a scrambling motion until fully cooked. Remove from the heat, add salt and pepper to taste, and enjoy with the roasted potatoes.

Nutritional Analysis: Calories 360, Total Fat 18 g, Saturated Fat 4 g, Cholesterol 430 mg, Sodium 310 mg, Carbohydrates 30 g, Dietary Fiber 5 g, Protein 19 g

Speedy Spinach Breakfast Tacos

Time: Prep: 15 minutes; Cook: 15 minutes
Serves 4

Tacos for breakfast? Sure, why not! Spinach, black beans, and avocado up the fiber content, while chili powder adds a nice little kick to the black beans; but omit it if you are sensitive to spice at the moment. For a heartier meal, use large whole wheat flour tortillas instead and make a breakfast burrito.

1 tablespoon olive oil

1 small yellow onion, diced

2 cups packed spinach

8 large eggs

8 corn tortillas

1 (15-ounce) can black beans, drained and rinsed

1 teaspoon chili powder (optional)

Salt and freshly ground black pepper

1 tomato, seeded and diced

1 ripe avocado, peeled, pitted, and diced

½ cup shredded Cheddar cheese (about 4 ounces) (optional)

1. Preheat the oven to 200°F.
2. In a large skillet, heat the olive oil over medium heat. Add the onion and sauté until translucent, for 3 to 5 minutes.
3. Add the spinach to the skillet and cook until just wilted, for about 2 minutes.
4. Crack the eggs into a bowl and beat well. Pour the eggs evenly over the vegetables and allow to cook for 1 minute. Using a spatula, start stirring the egg mixture so that everything stays clumped together. Cook for 2 to 5 minutes more, until the eggs are fully cooked and scrambled.
5. Meanwhile, wrap the tortillas in foil and put them in the preheated oven until warmed through, for about 7 minutes.
6. Heat the black beans with chili powder, if using, in a saucepan over medium-low heat until warmed through.
7. Remove the tortillas from their foil, add the black beans, scrambled eggs, and vegetables, and top with diced tomato and avocado. Sprinkle Cheddar cheese on top, if using, and enjoy.

Lack of Appetite +

Nausea, Vomiting, or Heartburn

Constipation +

Diarrhea

Fatigue +

Mouth Sores

Dry Mouth +

Chewing or Swallowing Difficulty +

Taste Aversion— Sweet

Taste Aversion— Sour & Bitter +

Lack of Taste +

Smells Bother

Nutritional Analysis (as prepared without the Cheddar cheese): Calories 437, Total Fat 21 g, Saturated Fat 5 g, Cholesterol 430 mg, Sodium 526 mg, Carbohydrates 42 g, Dietary Fiber 11 g, Protein 21 g

Nutritional Analysis (as prepared with 1 tablespoon [1 ounce] Cheddar cheese per serving): Calories 550, Total Fat 30 g, Saturated Fat 11 g, Cholesterol 459 mg, Sodium 700 mg, Carbohydrates 42 g, Dietary Fiber 11 g, Protein 28 g

Eggy Quinoa Patties ⓘ

Time: Prep: 15 minutes; Cook: 15 minutes
Serves 4

These patties are the perfect topper to a big salad or bed of sautéed garlicky greens. Cook the quinoa ahead of time so you can just stir together all of the ingredients quickly. The quinoa mixture keeps nicely in the refrigerator for a few days.

2½ cups cooked quinoa, chilled
  or at room temperature
2 large eggs
½ cup large egg whites
  (about 4 eggs)
2 scallions, finely chopped

¼ cup sharp Cheddar cheese
  (about 2 ounces)
½ teaspoon salt
¼ teaspoon freshly ground black pepper
1 cup bread crumbs
2 tablespoons olive oil

1. Combine the quinoa, eggs, egg whites, scallions, cheese, salt, and pepper in a medium-size bowl.
2. Add the bread crumbs, stir, and let sit for a few minutes so the bread crumbs can absorb some of the moisture. Form into eight patties.
3. Heat 1 tablespoon of the olive oil in a large skillet over medium-high heat.
4. Add four of the patties with some room between them and cook until the bottoms are deeply browned, for 7 to 10 minutes. Carefully flip the patties with a spatula and cook the second sides for 5 minutes more, or until golden. Repeat with the remaining tablespoon of olive oil and remaining four patties.
5. Transfer the cooked patties to a serving plate.

Nutritional Analysis: Calories 350, Total Fat 14 g, Saturated Fat 3 g, Cholesterol 115 mg, Sodium 409 mg, Carbohydrates 41 g, Dietary Fiber 4 g, Protein 15 g

Lack of Appetite +
Nausea, Vomiting, or Heartburn +
Constipation +
Diarrhea
Fatigue +
Mouth Sores +
Dry Mouth +
Chewing or Swallowing Difficulty +
Taste Aversion—Sweet
Taste Aversion—Sour & Bitter +
Lack of Taste +
Smells Bother +

Sweet or Savory Matzoh Brei ⓘ

Time: Prep: 10 minutes; Cook: 10 minutes
Serves 4

Lack of
Appetite

Nausea,
Vomiting, or
Heartburn

Constipation

Diarrhea

Fatigue

Mouth
Sores

Dry
Mouth

Chewing or
Swallowing
Difficulty

Taste
Aversion—
Sweet

Taste
Aversion—
Sour & Bitter

Lack of
Taste

Smells
Bother

Matzoh brei is a traditional dish made of matzoh panfried with eggs and it can be made sweet or savory. To make it sweet, add a few shakes of cinnamon and some fresh fruit. To make it savory, add vegetables, such as mushrooms or spinach, and serve with a dash of hot sauce. Matzoh crackers are a great snack when topped with a spread of cream cheese, peanut butter and jelly, or our Supersmooth Ginger Hummus (page 223). Or make matzoh pizza: top matzoh with pizza sauce and shredded cheese and heat in the microwave or toaster oven until the cheese melts.

6 large eggs
½ cup milk
4 sheets plain matzoh
2 tablespoons unsalted butter
Sweet option: drizzle of pure maple

syrup or honey, plus ground
cinnamon and fruit (optional)
Savory option: pinch of salt and freshly
ground black pepper, plus vegetables and hot sauce (optional)

1. Crack the eggs into a bowl. Add the milk and whisk until smooth.
2. Rinse the pieces of matzoh under cold water for about 10 seconds, or until they are slightly softened but can still hold their shape.
3. Break up the matzoh into small pieces (about 1 inch) and add to the egg mixture. With a wooden spoon, stir the egg mixture and make sure each piece of matzoh is well coated with egg. Let sit for about 1 minute.
4. Melt the butter in a skillet over medium-high heat. Once the butter begins to foam at the edges, add the matzoh mixture to the pan.
5. Lower the heat to medium-low and stir the egg mixture from time to time, scraping up the bits that have stuck to the bottom. The eggs should be done in roughly 5 to 7 minutes.
6. Serve as sweet or savory, as desired.

Nutritional Analysis (not including sweet or savory add-ins): Calories 279, Total Fat 13 g, Saturated Fat 6 g, Cholesterol 339 mg, Sodium 112 mg, Carbohydrates 27 g, Dietary Fiber 0 g, Protein 13 g

Cracked Eggs in Zucchini-Corn-Lime Sauté

Time: Prep: 10 minutes; Cook: 30 minutes
Serves 2

Try this fun twist on a "Toad in a Hole" that uses vegetables instead of bread to hold the egg. For added calories, use whole-milk ricotta cheese. Cook the yolk all the way through if following an antimicrobial diet (a special diet for those with a weakened immune system that helps protect from bacteria and other harmful organisms that may be found in some food and drinks). Reduce or omit lime as needed if sensitive to acidity.

1 tablespoon olive oil
½ small onion, diced
1 cup canned, fresh, or frozen sweet
    corn kernels (drained and rinsed
    if canned, thawed if frozen)
1 cup diced zucchini

Juice of ½ lime
¼ teaspoon salt
2 large eggs
To serve: part-skim ricotta cheese
    and fresh basil, or salsa and
    fresh cilantro

1. In a medium-size skillet, heat the olive oil over medium-low heat.
2. Add the onion to the skillet and sauté until translucent, for 6 to 8 minutes.
3. Stir in the corn kernels and zucchini and cook until tender, for 5 minutes more. Stir in the lime juice and salt.
4. Create two wells in the zucchini mixture and crack an egg into each well. Lower the heat to low, cover, and let cook until the egg yolks are set to your desired consistency, for 5 to 10 minutes.
5. Remove from the heat and serve with ricotta cheese and basil, or salsa and cilantro.

Nutritional Analysis (not including ricotta cheese, salsa, or herbs):
Calories 231, Total Fat 12 g, Saturated Fat 3 g, Cholesterol 215 mg, Sodium 365 mg, Carbohydrates 25 g, Dietary Fiber 3 g, Protein 10 g

Nutritional Analysis (includes 1 tablespoon part-skim ricotta cheese and 1 teaspoon fresh basil): Calories 254, Total Fat 14 g, Saturated Fat 4 g, Cholesterol 223 mg, Sodium 386 mg, Carbohydrates 26 g, Dietary Fiber 3 g, Protein 27 g

Lack of Appetite +

Nausea, Vomiting, or Heartburn

Constipation +

Diarrhea

Fatigue +

Mouth Sores

Dry Mouth +

Chewing or Swallowing Difficulty +

Taste Aversion— Sweet +

Taste Aversion— Sour & Bitter +

Lack of Taste +

Smells Bother +

Nutritional Analysis (includes 1 tablespoon salsa and 1 teaspoon fresh cilantro): Calories 236, Total Fat 12 g, Saturated Fat 3 g, Cholesterol 215 mg, Sodium 493 mg, Carbohydrates 26 g, Dietary Fiber 3 g, Protein 10 g

Cauliflower Crust Quiche

Time: Prep: 15 minutes; Cook: 1 hour 30 minutes
Serves 4 to 6

A cauliflower crust is a great solution for those looking to cut down on saturated fats, which are often found in pastry doughs. The soft texture of quiches are great for those with a sore mouth or chewing difficulty. Omit the black pepper if sensitive to spices. Try mixing a cup of chopped greens into the egg mixture, for added color and nutrients. Leftover slices can be kept in the refrigerator for 1 to 2 days.

1 medium-size head cauliflower (4 to 5 cups chopped)
½ cup grated Parmesan cheese
1 teaspoon minced fresh rosemary
5 large eggs

1 teaspoon olive oil
1 cup milk
½ teaspoon salt
½ teaspoon freshly ground black pepper

1. Preheat the oven to 375°F.
2. Pulse the cauliflower in the food processor until it resembles small couscous-size pieces. Alternatively, grate the cauliflower on a box grater.
3. Place the cauliflower into a microwave-safe dish and microwave it on high power for about 5 minutes, or until the cauliflower pieces are cooked. Let cool for about 10 minutes. Careful, it will be hot!
4. Dump the cauliflower into a clean kitchen towel, twist the towel closed, and squeeze out as much liquid as you can. Place the cauliflower back in the bowl and stir in the Parmesan cheese, rosemary, and one of the eggs.
5. Grease a 9-inch pie plate with the olive oil. Press the cauliflower mixture into the bottom and sides of the pie plate and heat in the oven for 15 to 20 minutes, until the mixture is warmed through and slightly golden. Let cool for 5 minutes.
6. While the crust bakes, whisk together the remaining four eggs, milk, salt, and pepper. Pour over the baked cauliflower crust. Return the pie plate to the oven and bake for 40 to 50 minutes more, or until the eggs are set (they should puff up and hardly jiggle).
7. Remove from the oven and let cool slightly before serving.

Lack of Appetite +

Nausea, Vomiting, or Heartburn

Constipation +

Diarrhea

Fatigue +

Mouth Sores +

Dry Mouth +

Chewing or Swallowing Difficulty +

Taste Aversion— Sweet

Taste Aversion— Sour & Bitter +

Lack of Taste +

Smells Bother +

Nutritional Analysis: Calories 181, Total Fat 10 g, Saturated Fat 4 g, Cholesterol 281 mg, Sodium 518 mg, Carbohydrates 8 g, Dietary Fiber 1 g, Protein 15 g

Sweet Potato, Tomato, and Spinach Hash ⓘ

Time: Prep: 15 minutes; Cook: 15 minutes
Serves 2

Red, orange, yellow, green, and . . . okay, maybe not blue, but you get the picture. Vitamins abound in this colorful hash and one feels healthier just for eating it. For added protein, add tofu, chicken, or turkey. Omit the tomatoes if experiencing mouth sores.

....

1 tablespoon + 1 teaspoon olive oil

1 cup finely diced sweet potato

2 small garlic cloves, minced

1 cup diced tomatoes

2 cups fresh spinach

2 large eggs

Salt and freshly ground
    black pepper
....

1. Heat 1 tablespoon of the olive oil in a skillet over medium heat.
2. Add the sweet potatoes and cook until tender, for 5 to 10 minutes. Add the garlic and cook for 30 seconds.
3. Stir in the tomatoes and cook for 2 minutes, then add the spinach and cook until just wilted.
4. Push the hash to one side of the pan to clear a space for the eggs. Add the remaining teaspoon of olive oil to the space, and then the eggs. Cook until the egg yolks reach your desired doneness— scrambled or sunny-side up both work well. Season with a pinch of salt and pepper and enjoy.

Nutritional Analysis: Calories 237, Total Fat 14 g, Saturated Fat 3 g, Cholesterol 215 mg, Sodium 385 mg, Carbohydrates 21 g, Dietary Fiber 4 g, Protein 9 g

Lack of Appetite +

Nausea, Vomiting, or Heartburn

Constipation +

Diarrhea

Fatigue +

Mouth Sores

Dry Mouth +

Chewing or Swallowing Difficulty +

Taste Aversion— Sweet

Taste Aversion— Sour & Bitter +

Lack of Taste +

Smells Bother

Tofu Scramble with Pesto and Roasted Cherry Tomatoes

Time: Prep: 10 minutes; Cook: 30 minutes
Serves 3

Lack of
Appetite

Nausea,
Vomiting, or
Heartburn

Constipation

Diarrhea

Fatigue

Mouth
Sores

Dry
Mouth

Chewing or
Swallowing
Difficulty

Taste
Aversion—
Sweet

Taste
Aversion—
Sour & Bitter

Lack of
Taste

Smells
Bother

Our zesty basil pesto pairs beautifully with tofu and tomatoes in this vegetarian breakfast scramble. But for those egg lovers, the tofu can easily be replaced with eggs. For a bigger breakfast, serve with yogurt and blueberries, or with a big side of Sweet Potato Home Fries (page 193). Reduce the garlic and onion as needed if sensitive to aromatics.

1 (14-ounce) block firm or extra-firm tofu
1 pint cherry or grape tomatoes, sliced in half
1 tablespoon + 2 teaspoons olive oil
Pinch each of salt and freshly ground

black pepper
1 small onion, chopped
1 garlic clove, minced
¼ cup prepared Basic Pesto (page 219)

1. Press the extra water out of the tofu: Wrap the tofu with a few layers of paper towel and place on a plate. Place another plate on top and add a heavy can on top of this to give the tofu a good "pressing." Let sit for at least 10 to 20 minutes to soak out most of the water.
2. Preheat the oven to 450°F. Toss the tomatoes with 2 teaspoons of the olive oil and the salt and pepper and place on a baking sheet. Roast for 15 to 20 minutes, or until the tomatoes are soft and just starting to wrinkle.
3. While the tomatoes are roasting, heat the remaining tablespoon of olive oil in a skillet over medium heat.
4. Add the chopped onion and cook for about 5 minutes, until the onion is translucent and shiny, then add the garlic and cook for another 2 minutes.
5. Crumble in the pressed tofu and sauté for about 10 minutes, stirring frequently. (Cook longer if the tofu is still mushy.)
6. Add the pesto and cook for 2 minutes. Remove from the heat and top with roasted tomatoes.

Nutritional Analysis: Calories 300, Total Fat 23 g, Saturated Fat 3 g, Cholesterol 1 mg, Sodium 136 mg, Carbohydrates 11 g, Dietary Fiber 3 g, Protein 15 g

Nutritionist's Favorite to Savor ··

This recipe is my favorite because it integrates pesto into the morning meal. For those experiencing flavor fatigue, don't be afraid to go out of your flavor comfort zone here. Pesto adds a serious punch to a basic tofu scramble.

Seitan, Apple, and Broccoli Breakfast Hash ◑

Time: Prep: 15 minutes; Cook: 15 minutes
Serves 2

Lack of
Appetite

Nausea,
Vomiting, or
Heartburn

Constipation

Diarrhea

Fatigue

Mouth
Sores

Dry
Mouth

Chewing or
Swallowing
Difficulty

Taste
Aversion—
Sweet

Taste
Aversion—
Sour & Bitter

Lack of
Taste

Smells
Bother

This savory hash sneaks in some sweet tones from the apple and is a great way to get one serving of vegetables, fruit, and protein in one meal. Add a slice of whole wheat bread and the grains are covered, too. You may substitute tempeh for the seitan. Both seitan and tempeh are vegetarian proteins that mimic the taste and mouthfeel of common animal proteins. If animal protein is desired, try chopped lean turkey or chicken.

2 to 3 teaspoons olive oil

5 ounces cooked seitan, chopped

1 apple, cored and cut into small cubes

1 cup broccoli florets

2 scallions, chopped

2 tablespoons raw cashews

Salt and freshly ground black pepper

2 large eggs

1. Heat 1 to 2 teaspoons of the oil in a medium-size nonstick skillet over medium heat.
2. Add the pieces of seitan and cook until golden brown, for 3 to 5 minutes.
3. Add the apples and cook until softened, for about 2 minutes.
4. Meanwhile, place the broccoli in a small bowl and add 1 tablespoon of water. Cover with an extra, microwave-safe plate and cook in the microwave on high power for 1 minute. Remove, drain the water, and add the broccoli to the seitan mixture. Stir in the scallions and cashews, adjust the seasoning, and continue to cook for about 30 seconds. Transfer to a plate and set aside.
5. Return the skillet to the heat, add more oil if necessary, and panfry the eggs to your desired yolk doneness. Carefully place the fried eggs over the seitan mixture and serve immediately.

Nutritional Analysis: Calories 400, Total Fat 18 g, Saturated Fat 3 g, Cholesterol 215 mg, Sodium 536 mg, Carbohydrates 32 g, Dietary Fiber 4 g, Protein 33 g

Vegan Mushroom Breakfast Burritos

Time: Prep: 30 minutes; Cook: 30 minutes
Serves 4

Nutritional yeast is a good source of B vitamins and nonvegans can easily replace the tofu with eggs, which are also a good source of B vitamins. Save leftovers in the refrigerator for up to 2 days. Serve with a side of black beans for added fiber.

1 (14-ounce) package firm or
  extra-firm tofu
2 tablespoons olive oil
2 potatoes, finely diced
1 medium-size onion, diced
1½ cups sliced mushrooms
2 garlic cloves, minced
½ teaspoon ground turmeric

½ teaspoon paprika
¼ cup nutritional yeast
2 tablespoons chopped fresh basil
Salt and freshly ground black pepper
4 (8-inch) whole wheat tortillas
Salsa, for topping
Chopped scallions, for topping
  (optional)

1. Press the extra water out of the tofu: Wrap the tofu with a few layers of paper towel and place on a plate. Place another plate on top and add a heavy can on top of this to give the tofu a good "pressing." Let sit for at least 10 to 20 minutes to soak out most of the water.
2. Meanwhile, heat 1 tablespoon of the oil in a large, nonstick skillet over medium heat, add the potatoes, and sauté until tender and golden brown, for 10 to 15 minutes. Transfer the potatoes to a bowl.
3. To the skillet, add the remaining tablespoon of oil and sauté the onion until translucent.
4. Add the mushrooms and garlic and cook for another 3 to 5 minutes, until the mushrooms are cooked down.
5. Remove the tofu from the towels and dice it finely.
6. Lower the heat to low and stir in the diced tofu, turmeric, paprika, nutritional yeast, basil, and potatoes. Cook until the tofu is warmed through. Season with salt and pepper to taste.
7. Divide the mixture among four tortilla wraps, spoon on salsa, and top with chopped scallions, if desired.

Lack of Appetite	+
Nausea, Vomiting, or Heartburn	
Constipation	+
Diarrhea	
Fatigue	+
Mouth Sores	+
Dry Mouth	+
Chewing or Swallowing Difficulty	+
Taste Aversion— Sweet	
Taste Aversion— Sour & Bitter	+
Lack of Taste	+
Smells Bother	

Nutritional Analysis (not including salsa or scallions): Calories 339, Total Fat 14 g, Saturated Fat 2 g, Cholesterol 0 mg, Sodium 367 mg, Carbohydrates 36 g, Dietary Fiber 8 g, Protein 19 g

Chicken, Apple, and Maple Breakfast Patties

Time: Prep: 15 minutes; Cook: 30 minutes
Makes 16 small patties

This classic flavor combination will have you including this recipe in regular rotation. Try it with a pinch of nutmeg and/or cinnamon for a variation. Reduce the garlic and pepper as needed for taste sensitivity. Store leftover patties in the refrigerator for up to 2 days or in the freezer for up to 1 month.

1 teaspoon olive oil	¼ cup all-purpose flour
½ medium-size leek, finely chopped	1½ tablespoons pure maple syrup
1 garlic clove, minced	2 large egg whites
1 apple, cored and finely chopped	½ teaspoon salt
1 pound ground chicken breast	¼ teaspoon freshly ground black pepper

1. Preheat the oven to 450°F. Line a large baking sheet with parchment paper and set aside.
2. Heat the olive oil in a large pan over medium heat.
3. Add the leek and garlic and cook until the garlic becomes fragrant, for about 2 minutes.
4. Add the diced apple and cook for a few minutes more, or until the apple softens. Remove from the heat, transfer to a large bowl, and let cool for 2 minutes.
5. Mix the ground chicken with the sautéed leek mixture. Mix in the flour to coat.
6. In a small bowl, whisk together the maple syrup and egg whites. Stir into the chicken mixture.
7. Divide into sixteen small patties and place on the prepared baking sheet. Bake for 20 to 25 minutes, or until the patties are completely cooked through and the outside has browned.

Nutritional Analysis (per patty): Calories 65, Total Fat 3 g, Saturated Fat 1 g, Cholesterol 24 mg, Sodium 85 mg, Carbohydrates 5 g, Dietary Fiber 0 g, Protein 6 g

Lack of Appetite +
Nausea, Vomiting, or Heartburn +
Constipation +
Diarrhea +
Fatigue +
Mouth Sores +
Dry Mouth +
Chewing or Swallowing Difficulty +
Taste Aversion— Sweet
Taste Aversion— Sour & Bitter +
Lack of Taste +
Smells Bother

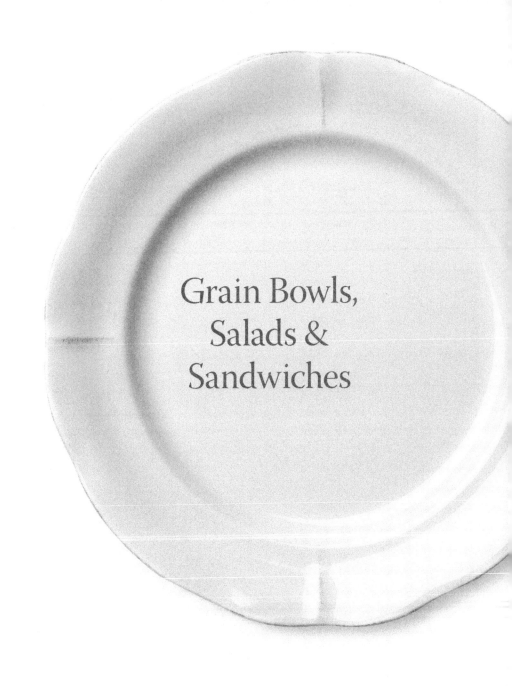

Grain Bowls,
Salads &
Sandwiches

Quinoa Bowl with Sliced Avocado and Yogurt Dressing ⓘ

Time: Prep: 15 minutes; Cook: 15 minutes
Serves 4 to 6

Lack of Appetite

Nausea, Vomiting, or Heartburn

Constipation

Diarrhea

Fatigue

Mouth Sores

Dry Mouth

Chewing or Swallowing Difficulty

Taste Aversion—Sweet

Taste Aversion—Sour & Bitter

Lack of Taste

Smells Bother

A hearty bowl of protein packed quinoa, fresh greens, healthy fats, and a generous dollop of zesty tang. Yes, please! Crush or omit the almonds if experiencing chewing difficulty. Try adding your favorite beans, for extra protein and fiber.

1 cup uncooked quinoa

2 cups arugula or spinach

3 ounces pasteurized Cotija, feta, or ricotta salata cheese

½ cup toasted almonds or a mix of seeds and nuts

¼ teaspoon salt, or to taste

1 ripe avocado, pitted, peeled, and thinly sliced

For the dressing

1 cup plain yogurt

Zest of ½ lemon

½ tablespoon freshly squeezed lemon juice

2 tablespoons chopped fresh chives, plus more for serving

⅛ teaspoon salt

1. Rinse the quinoa in a fine-mesh sieve under running water. Place in a saucepan with 2 cups of water and bring to a boil. Lower the heat to low, cover, and simmer for about 15 minutes, until the water is absorbed and tiny spirals start to separate from and curl around the quinoa seeds. Turn off the heat, fluff the quinoa with a fork, and let it cool to room temperature, for at least 20 minutes.
2. In a large bowl, combine the cooled quinoa, arugula, cheese, almonds, and salt. Mix well. Top the salad with the avocado slices.
3. Make the yogurt dressing by whisking together the yogurt, lemon zest and juice, chives, and salt in a small bowl.
4. Serve the salad with big dollops of yogurt dressing and extra chopped chives.

Nutritional Analysis (includes salad and dressing together): Calories 448, Total Fat 25 g, Saturated Fat 5 g, Cholesterol 18 mg, Sodium 445 mg, Carbohydrates 42 g, Dietary Fiber 9 g, Protein 18 g

Very Veggie Farro Salad

Time: Prep: 15 minutes; Cook: 1 hour
Serves 4

This salad can be made with any whole grain you have on hand, but farro gives a nutty, chewy texture that's hard to resist. High fiber content from the whole grain and snap peas can help ease constipation. Leftover salad makes a great lunch on the second day. For extra protein, add a handful of beans or some grilled chicken.

1 cup uncooked farro

2 cups cherry or grape tomatoes

2 cups trimmed sugar snap peas

2 tablespoons olive oil

Salt and freshly ground black pepper

1 tablespoon unsalted butter

1 medium-size red onion, sliced

8 ounces white portobello mushrooms, sliced

2 tablespoons red wine vinegar

1. Cook the farro according to the package directions.
2. Meanwhile, preheat the oven to 400°F and line a baking sheet with parchment paper.
3. Place the tomatoes and snap peas in a single layer on the prepared baking sheet and evenly coat with 1 tablespoon of the olive oil. Sprinkle with salt and pepper and roast for 15 to 20 minutes, or until the tomatoes start to split.
4. In a skillet, melt the butter and remaining tablespoon of olive oil over medium heat. Add the sliced onion and mushrooms to the skillet. Let cook for 5 to 10 minutes.
5. Remove from the heat and add the red wine vinegar and a sprinkle of salt and pepper. Return the skillet to the heat and cook for another 5 minutes, or until everything is browned and deliciously caramelized.
6. Toss together the farro, tomatoes, snap peas, and mushroom mixture in a big bowl and enjoy.

Nutritional Analysis: Calories 325, Total Fat 10 g, Saturated Fat 3 g, Cholesterol 8 mg, Sodium 254 mg, Carbohydrates 51 g, Dietary Fiber 11 g, Protein 8 g

Lack of Appetite +

Nausea, Vomiting, or Heartburn

Constipation +

Diarrhea

Fatigue +

Mouth Sores

Dry Mouth +

Chewing or Swallowing Difficulty

Taste Aversion— Sweet +

Taste Aversion— Sour & Bitter

Lack of Taste +

Smells Bother

Warm Lima Bean and Asparagus Salad with Arugula Parsley Pesto

Time: Prep: 15 minutes; Cook: 30 minutes
Serves 6

Lack of
Appetite

Nausea,
Vomiting, or
Heartburn

Constipation

Diarrhea

Fatigue

Mouth
Sores

Dry
Mouth

Chewing or
Swallowing
Difficulty

Taste
Aversion—
Sweet

Taste
Aversion—
Sour & Bitter

Lack of
Taste

Smells
Bother

Four shades of green. And who says greens aren't exciting? Finally, the oft-underutilized lima bean makes an appearance, bringing protein, fiber, and a variety of minerals to the table. Now *this* is our idea of a green salad!

1 bunch asparagus
½ cup + 2 teaspoons olive oil
Salt
1 cup frozen lima beans
4 cups arugula
½ cup fresh parsley

1 garlic clove, peeled
1 tablespoon balsamic vinegar
Zest and juice of 1 lemon
Freshly ground black pepper
2 tablespoons shaved Pecorino Romano
   or Parmesan cheese

1. Preheat the oven to 400°F. Cut the asparagus into 1-inch pieces and place on a baking sheet. Drizzle with 2 teaspoons of the olive oil and sprinkle with ¼ teaspoon of salt. Roast for about 10 minutes, or until the asparagus has turned bright green and is slightly charred and roasted.
2. Meanwhile, bring a saucepan of water to a boil. Add the lima beans and simmer until tender but not mushy, for 5 to 10 minutes. Drain.
3. While the lima beans cook, put 2 cups of arugula and the parsley, the remaining ½ cup of oil, and the garlic, balsamic vinegar, lemon zest and juice, and a hearty pinch of salt and pepper in the bowl of a food processor or blender. Process until smooth like a pesto. Taste and add more salt or an extra squeeze of lemon juice, if needed.
4. Place the asparagus, lima beans, and remaining 2 cups of arugula in a bowl and toss together with the pesto. Top with the cheese.

Nutritional Analysis: Calories 234, Total Fat 20 g, Saturated Fat 3 g, Cholesterol 1 mg, Sodium 203 mg, Carbohydrates 10 g, Dietary Fiber 4 g, Protein 5 g

Thai-Style Vegetable Strand Salad ⓘ

Time: 30 minutes
Serves 2

Raw zucchini may seem strange at first, but its surprisingly tender skin and flesh is perfect in this flavorful dish. Of course, if more tender veggies are desired, they can always be steamed ahead of time. Sauté the veggies in a bit of oil, without the sauce, if averse to strong flavors. Doubling up on chickpeas or adding cooked tofu or chicken make wonderful additions, if extra protein is desired.

1 zucchini, cut into thin slices, julienned, or spiralized

2 carrots, cut into thin slices or spiralized

4 cups baby spinach, whole or roughly chopped

1 scallion, chopped

⅔ cup cooked chickpeas (drained and rinsed, if using canned)

2 tablespoons chopped cashews or peanuts, or toasted sesame seeds

For the dressing

Juice of 1 lime or lemon

1 garlic clove, finely minced

2 tablespoons peanut butter or nut butter of choice

2 teaspoons low-sodium soy sauce

1 teaspoon honey or agave nectar

1. In a large bowl, combine the zucchini, carrots, spinach, scallion, and chickpeas.
2. Combine all the dressing ingredients in a small bowl or cup, slowly adding up to 1 tablespoon of water to thin, if desired. Taste and adjust the ingredients as needed.
3. Add the dressing to the vegetables and mix thoroughly.
4. Transfer to plates and top with the chopped nuts or seeds.

Nutritional Analysis: Calories 325, Total Fat 16 g, Saturated Fat 3 g, Cholesterol 0 mg, Sodium 385 mg, Carbohydrates 39 g, Dietary Fiber 10 g, Protein 14 g

Lack of Appetite +

Nausea, Vomiting, or Heartburn

Constipation +

Diarrhea

Fatigue +

Mouth Sores

Dry Mouth +

Chewing or Swallowing Difficulty

Taste Aversion— Sweet +

Taste Aversion— Sour & Bitter

Lack of Taste +

Smells Bother +

Carrot, Date, and Chickpea Salad ⓘ

Time: 30 minutes

Serves 6

This salad is all about textures—crunchy carrots, soft dates, and firm chickpeas. It's a playground for your mouth. Don't worry if you need to steam the carrots for a softer texture; the cumin dressing adds another layer of fun all on its own. Toss leftovers over your favorite greens for a salad the next day. For added protein, add hard-boiled egg, chicken, or turkey.

⅓ cup olive oil

2 tablespoons freshly squeezed
lemon juice

1 teaspoon honey

1 tablespoon ground cumin

½ teaspoon salt, plus
more to taste

⅛ teaspoon cayenne pepper

10 ounces carrots (about 4 large),
shredded

1 (15-ounce) can chickpeas,
drained and rinsed

⅔ cup dates, pitted and cut
into 1-inch pieces

⅓ cup fresh mint, torn

1 tablespoon toasted almond slices

1. In a bowl or jar, whisk together the olive oil, lemon juice, honey, cumin, salt, and cayenne. Set aside.
2. In a separate bowl, combine the carrots, chickpeas, dates, mint, and almonds.
3. Gently toss until everything is evenly coated.
4. Serve immediately, or cover and refrigerate until ready to serve.

Nutritional Analysis: Calories 265, Total Fat 14 g, Saturated Fat 2 g, Cholesterol 0 mg, Sodium 339 mg, Carbohydrates 35 g, Dietary Fiber 4 g, Protein 5 g

Lack of
Appetite

Nausea,
Vomiting, or
Heartburn

Constipation

Diarrhea

Fatigue

Mouth
Sores

Dry
Mouth

Chewing or
Swallowing
Difficulty

Taste
Aversion—
Sweet

Taste
Aversion—
Sour & Bitter

Lack of
Taste

Smells
Bother

Drunken Feta Caprese Salad ◖

Time: Prep: 10 minutes + 5 hours resting
Serves 4

Aged balsamic vinegar is thicker and sweeter than regular balsamic vinegar and therefore worth seeking out for this intoxicatingly delicious recipe. It can also be made into an entrée by mixing in a whole grain, couscous, or pasta. Alternatively, make a grilled panini sandwich by stuffing a ciabatta or baguette and heating it on the stovetop or in the oven to melt the cheese.

....

8 medium-size plum tomatoes, chopped into 1-inch pieces

1 large bunch fresh basil, finely chopped

1½ cups crumbled pasteurized feta cheese

¼ to ½ cup aged balsamic vinegar (the more vinegar, the "drunker" the salad)

Pinch of salt

....

Mix all the ingredients together. Let sit in the refrigerator for at least 5 hours for the balsamic to really soak into the ingredients. Remove from the refrigerator 30 minutes before serving.

Nutritional Analysis: Calories 189, Total Fat 12 g, Saturated Fat 8 g, Cholesterol 50 mg, Sodium 711 mg, Carbohydrates 10 g, Dietary Fiber 2 g, Protein 10 g

Lack of Appetite	+
Nausea, Vomiting, or Heartburn	
Constipation	+
Diarrhea	
Fatigue	+
Mouth Sores	
Dry Mouth	+
Chewing or Swallowing Difficulty	+
Taste Aversion— Sweet	+
Taste Aversion— Sour & Bitter	
Lack of Taste	+
Smells Bother	

Summery Black Bean, Jicama, and Corn Salad ⓘ

Time: 15 minutes
Serves 6

Lack of
Appetite

Nausea,
Vomiting, or
Heartburn

Constipation

Diarrhea

Fatigue

Mouth
Sores

Dry
Mouth

Chewing or
Swallowing
Difficulty

Taste
Aversion—
Sweet

Taste
Aversion—
Sour & Bitter

Lack of
Taste

Smells
Bother

Try it grilled—corn has a great smoky flavor when grilled, adding more depth and flavor to the salad. If you don't have a grill, sauté the corn in a pan with some olive oil over medium heat, stirring occasionally, letting the kernels get golden brown. Stuff leftovers into a taco, burrito, or pita pocket. Or serve the salad atop a piece of mild white fish.

2 (15-ounce) cans black beans,
   drained and rinsed
4 medium-size cobs, kernels
   shaved off the cob (about 4 cups)
1 large jicama, peeled and chopped into

1-inch pieces
1 large bunch fresh cilantro, chopped
Juice of 1 lime
Salt and freshly ground black pepper
Olive oil (optional)

1. Mix together the black beans, corn, jicama, and cilantro. Squirt with lime juice and sprinkle with salt and pepper to taste. Add a drizzle of olive oil, if desired.

Nutritional Analysis: Calories 256, Total Fat 1 g, Saturated Fat 0 g, Cholesterol 0 mg, Sodium 187 mg, Carbohydrates 54 g, Dietary Fiber 17 g, Protein 11 g

Red Cabbage Slaw with
Pecans and Double Citrus Dressing ◑

Time: 30 minutes

Serves 8

This sweet and crunchy cabbage slaw adds an exciting element to a sandwich. Or enjoy alongside baked beans and corn bread for a southern variation. Grated carrots work well instead of or in addition to the cabbage. Also consider swapping out a quarter of the cabbage for matchstick apple slices from one apple. To tone down the acidity in the dressing, replace the lemon juice with ½ cup plain Greek yogurt.

1 head red cabbage, shredded	2 tablespoons honey
1 cup pecans, toasted and	2 tablespoons olive oil
chopped	Salt and freshly ground black pepper
Juice of ½ orange	Chopped fresh cilantro or mint,
Juice of ½ lemon	for garnish

1. Combine the cabbage and pecans in a large bowl.
2. Whisk together the remaining ingredients, except the fresh herbs, and toss with the cabbage and pecans.
3. Refrigerate for at least 30 minutes so the flavors can blend. Garnish with the herbs and serve.

Nutritional Analysis: Calories 128, Total Fat 8 g, Saturated Fat 1 g, Cholesterol 0 mg, Sodium 149 mg, Carbohydrates 14 g, Dietary Fiber 3 g, Protein 2 g

Symptom	
Lack of Appetite	+
Nausea, Vomiting, or Heartburn	
Constipation	+
Diarrhea	
Fatigue	+
Mouth Sores	
Dry Mouth	+
Chewing or Swallowing Difficulty	
Taste Aversion—Sweet	
Taste Aversion—Sour & Bitter	+
Lack of Taste	+
Smells Bother	

Creamy Avocado Egg Salad ⓘ

Time: Prep: 10 minutes; Cook: 7 minutes
Serves 6

Lack of Appetite

Nausea, Vomiting, or Heartburn

Constipation

Diarrhea

Fatigue

Mouth Sores

Dry Mouth

Chewing or Swallowing Difficulty

Taste Aversion— Sweet

Taste Aversion— Sour & Bitter

Lack of Taste

Smells Bother

A creamy protein-packed salad with wonderful mouthfeel, this makes for a hearty lunch or snack any day. Omit the vinegar and onion in the dressing if you have mouth sores.

6 large hard-boiled eggs, chopped
1½ medium-size avocados, peeled, pitted, and cubed
2 tablespoons plain Greek yogurt or mayonnaise

1 tablespoon finely chopped red onion
2 teaspoons red wine vinegar
½ teaspoon salt
Pinch of freshly ground black pepper

1. In a bowl, combine all the ingredients.
2. Mash slightly with a fork.
3. Enjoy atop a salad, toast, or crackers.

Nutritional Analysis: Calories 243, Total Fat 19 g, Saturated Fat 4 g, Cholesterol 280 mg, Sodium 341 mg, Carbohydrates 8 g, Dietary Fiber 5 g, Protein 12 g

Nutritionist's Favorite to Savor
This is my favorite because the avocado and egg ingredients are nutritionally dense, meaning they provide good calories, protein, and vitamins and minerals, and the avocado adds healthy monounsaturated fat. Nutrient dense foods are both good for someone trying to gain weight and for someone trying to lose or maintain weight.

Chicken Salad with Celery and Grapes

Time: Prep: 30 minutes; Cook: 10 minutes
Serves 4

This bright and colorful salad is cool and refreshing and gets better overnight so consider setting some aside for lunch the next day. If you like nuts, chopped walnuts, almonds, or pecans would be a wonderful addition to this recipe. For vegetarian options, use cubed tofu or tempeh instead of chicken.

....

2 medium-size boneless, skinless
   chicken breasts
Salt and freshly ground black pepper
1 teaspoon chili powder
1 tablespoon olive oil
½ cup diced celery

1 cup red grapes, halved
1 medium-size carrot, diced
2 tablespoons minced red onion
5 tablespoons plain Greek yogurt
Juice and zest of ½ lemon
½ cup fresh tarragon, chopped

....

1. Season the chicken breasts with salt, pepper, and the chili powder.
2. Heat the olive oil in a skillet over medium-high heat. Cook the chicken in the skillet until cooked through and brown on both sides, about 4 minutes per side. Remove from the heat. After the chicken has cooled, dice or shred into small pieces.
3. Toss the chopped celery, grapes, carrot, red onion, and cooled chicken together in a large bowl.
4. In a separate bowl, mix together Greek yogurt and the lemon juice and zest. Season with salt and pepper. Add the tarragon.
5. Toss the salad with the dressing and serve in a lettuce cup, as a sandwich, or with crackers.

Nutritional Analysis: Calories 158, Total Fat 5 g, Saturated Fat 1 g, Cholesterol 39 mg, Sodium 227 mg, Carbohydrates 11 g, Dietary Fiber 1 g, Protein 15 g

Lack of Appetite	+
Nausea, Vomiting, or Heartburn	+
Constipation	+
Diarrhea	
Fatigue	+
Mouth Sores	
Dry Mouth	+
Chewing or Swallowing Difficulty	
Taste Aversion—Sweet	
Taste Aversion—Sour & Bitter	+
Lack of Taste	+
Smells Bother	+

Double Cheese and Corn Quesadillas

Time: Prep: 10 minutes; Cook: 30 minutes

Serves 2

Lack of
Appetite

Nausea,
Vomiting, or
Heartburn

Constipation

Diarrhea

Fatigue

Mouth
Sores

Dry
Mouth

Chewing or
Swallowing
Difficulty

Taste
Aversion—
Sweet

Taste
Aversion—
Sour & Bitter

Lack of
Taste

Smells
Bother

This one is for cheese lovers. Jack and goat cheese are suggested, but feel free to use two of your favorite cheeses. For extra protein, try it with shredded or diced chicken or turkey, firm tofu, scrambled eggs, or the traditional black beans. For those sensitive to digesting corn, you can easily replace with any of your favorite beans or vegetables.

1½ cups fresh or frozen corn kernels

2 teaspoons olive oil

½ medium-size white onion

1 teaspoon olive oil, to grill the
quesadillas

2 (10-inch) flour tortillas

¼ cup grated Jack cheese

2 ounces pasteurized chèvre or other
pasteurized soft goat cheese or
cream cheese

1. Heat a large skillet over medium-high heat and place the corn kernels in the skillet. Cook, stirring and shaking frequently, until the kernels are slightly browned and smell fragrant (about 10 minutes). Transfer the corn to a plate and set aside.
2. Place the skillet back on the stove with 1 teaspoon of the olive oil, and heat over medium-high heat. Add the onion and cook, stirring occasionally, while the onion softens and browns, for about 5 minutes. Place on the plate with the corn.
3. Place the skillet back on the stove with ½ teaspoon of the olive oil over medium heat. Lay one tortilla in the pan.
4. Sprinkle one side of the tortilla with half of the Jack cheese.
5. Distribute half of the corn and half of the goat cheese over the Jack cheese, then fold the tortilla in half.
6. Make room in the skillet, add the remaining ½ teaspoon of oil, the second tortilla, and the remaining filling ingredients. Fold the tortilla over itself.
7. Cook the quesadillas until each side has browned, for 3 to 5 minutes per side. Cut into wedges and serve.

Nutritional Analysis: Calories 502, Total Fat 21 g, Saturated Fat 9 g, Cholesterol 28 mg, Sodium 787 mg, Carbohydrates 66 g, Dietary Fiber 5 g, Protein 19 g

Loaded Mozzarella Grilled Cheese ⓘ

Time: Prep: 5 minutes; Cook: 10 minutes
Serves 1

Cook this unique version of a grilled cheese sandwich in the classic way—on the stovetop, with butter for a nice brown crust on the bread. Be sure to press it down gently to get the ingredients to stick to the cheese. Hint: For a good "flip," support the top of the sandwich with your free hand while flipping. Use a soft bread or cut the crust off the bread if you have trouble chewing or swallowing.

1 teaspoon olive oil or unsalted butter	¼ avocado, peeled, pitted, and thinly sliced
2 slices sandwich bread	1 handful arugula
2 slices mozzarella cheese	2 slices tomato

1. Heat a skillet over medium heat and place the oil in the skillet.
2. Assemble the sandwich and place it in the skillet. Cook for about 4 minutes on each side, or until the cheese starts to melt and the bread starts to crisp up.

Nutritional Analysis: Calories 491, Total Fat 25 g, Saturated Fat 8 g, Cholesterol 20 mg, Sodium 623 mg, Carbohydrates 44 g, Dietary Fiber 10 g, Protein 25 g

Symptom	
Lack of Appetite	+
Nausea, Vomiting, or Heartburn	
Constipation	+
Diarrhea	
Fatigue	+
Mouth Sores	+
Dry Mouth	+
Chewing or Swallowing Difficulty	+
Taste Aversion—Sweet	+
Taste Aversion—Sour & Bitter	+
Lack of Taste	+
Smells Bother	+

Vegetable Pita Pizzas ①

Time: Prep: 10 minutes; Cook: 20 minutes
Serves 2

Lack of
Appetite

Nausea,
Vomiting, or
Heartburn

Constipation

Diarrhea

Fatigue

Mouth
Sores

Dry
Mouth

Chewing or
Swallowing
Difficulty

Taste
Aversion—
Sweet

Taste
Aversion—
Sour & Bitter

Lack of
Taste

Smells
Bother

Warm pita pizzas make a great snack or a light meal on any day. For more vegetables, serve alongside a salad. Try adding cooked chopped chicken, for extra protein. If looking for more flavor, add some anchovies. Their omega-3 fats and calcium make them a healthy addition to pizza.

½ tablespoon olive oil

2 (6-inch) whole wheat pita breads

⅔ cup Mirepoix Marinara Sauce
   (page 217)

½ cup shredded mozzarella cheese

1 cup thinly sliced vegetables, such as
   mushrooms, onion, or bell peppers

¼ cup fresh basil leaves, torn

1. Preheat the oven to 350°F.
2. Rub a baking sheet with the olive oil and place the pita breads on top.
3. Spread the marinara over the two pita breads and sprinkle with the shredded cheese.
4. Top with the sliced vegetables.
5. Place the baking sheet in the oven and bake for 15 to 20 minutes, or until the cheese is melted and the vegetables begin to wilt. Top with the basil.
6. Let the pita pizzas cool slightly, then transfer to a cutting board and cut into wedges.

Nutritional Analysis: Calories 321, Total Fat 12 g, Saturated Fat 4 g, Cholesterol 15 mg, Sodium 523 mg, Carbohydrates 44 g, Dietary Fiber 6 g, Protein 16 g

Lemony Chickpeas with Parsley ①

Time: 10 minutes
Serves 6

Enjoy this recipe as a side salad or a snack with homemade pita chips. Slice whole wheat pita bread into triangle wedges, drizzle with olive oil, place on a baking sheet, and bake in a 350°F oven for 10 to 15 minutes, until warmed and slightly crunchy. Yum! Leftover chickpeas can be pureed to spread on sandwiches or used as a dip for veggies or with the homemade pita chips.

2 (15-ounce) cans chickpeas, drained and rinsed	¼ teaspoon garlic powder
½ large red onion, finely diced	Juice of 2 lemons
1 teaspoon olive oil	½ large bunch flat-leaf parsley, chopped
¼ teaspoon ground cumin	Pinch of salt

Mix all the ingredients together. Enjoy.

Nutritional Analysis: Calories 135, Total Fat 3 g, Saturated Fat 0 g, Cholesterol 0 mg, Sodium 212 mg, Carbohydrates 22 g, Dietary Fiber 0 g, Protein 6 g

Lack of Appetite	+
Nausea, Vomiting, or Heartburn	
Constipation	+
Diarrhea	
Fatigue	+
Mouth Sores	
Dry Mouth	+
Chewing or Swallowing Difficulty	+
Taste Aversion— Sweet	+
Taste Aversion— Sour & Bitter	
Lack of Taste	+
Smells Bother	

Chickpea Salad Wraps
with Toasted Pumpkin Seeds

Time: Prep: 15 minutes; Cook: 10 minutes
Serves 4

Lack of
Appetite

Nausea,
Vomiting, or
Heartburn

Constipation

Diarrhea

Fatigue

Mouth
Sores

Dry
Mouth

Chewing or
Swallowing
Difficulty

Taste
Aversion—
Sweet

Taste
Aversion—
Sour & Bitter

Lack of
Taste

Smells
Bother

A different way to highlight the humble chickpea. Pumpkin seeds are a good source of magnesium and toasting them adds a lovely layer of flavor to the mixture. The chickpea mixture can be stored in the refrigerator for up to 5 days; just give it a stir before serving. Spread leftover chickpeas onto a piece of crunchy toast for a simple tartine. Omit the pumpkin seeds if experiencing gas, bloating, or lower digestive discomfort.

¼ cup pumpkin seeds

1 (15-ounce) can chickpeas, drained and rinsed

½ cup chopped celery

2 tablespoons chopped red onion

3 tablespoons chopped dill pickle (from about 1 pickle)

1 tablespoon chopped fresh dill

½ garlic clove, minced

½ teaspoon Dijon mustard

2 tablespoons freshly squeezed lemon juice

1 tablespoon olive oil

Salt and freshly ground black pepper

4 whole wheat wraps

1. Toast the pumpkin seeds in a dry skillet for about 5 minutes, or until just starting to smell fragrant and brown.
2. Mix the chickpeas, celery, red onion, pickle, dill, and garlic in a bowl, mashing up the chickpeas slightly with a fork. Stir in the toasted pumpkin seeds.
3. In a separate small bowl, whisk together the mustard, lemon juice, and olive oil and stir into the salad. Season with salt and pepper to taste.
4. Divide the salad among the four whole wheat wraps and roll each wrap up.

Nutritional Analysis: Calories 288, Total Fat 11 g, Saturated Fat 2 g, Cholesterol 0 mg, Sodium 561 mg, Carbohydrates 37 g, Dietary Fiber 4 g, Protein 11 g

Hummus and Cucumber Tartine ⓘ

Time: Prep: 5 minutes; Cook: 5 minutes
Serves 1

This is a great light meal for those looking to consume small, frequent meals to manage symptoms and improve nutritional intake. For a little extra flavor, give a light drizzle of balsamic vinegar on top. Try different types of breads to make the sandwich feel new again—whole wheat, sourdough, olive bread, and nut bread all pair well with hummus. Or swap out the bread for a pita or a wrap.

2 slices bread	2 thick slices tomato
4 tablespoons Supersmooth Ginger Hummus (page 223)	¼ cup cucumber slices
	¼ red onion, thinly sliced
2 slices Swiss cheese	Freshly ground pepper

1. Toast the bread in a toaster.
2. Spread each slice of toasted bread with hummus and top with a slice of cheese. Add the tomato, cucumber, and red onion slices and grind some pepper over the top. Enjoy.
3. Optional: Warm the tartine in a preheated 300°F toaster oven or an oven for about 5 minutes, just until the cheese melts.

Nutritional Analysis: Calories 554, Total Fat 25 g, Saturated Fat 12 g, Cholesterol 52 mg, Sodium 652 mg, Carbohydrates 53 g, Dietary Fiber 11 g, Protein 32 g

Lack of Appetite	+
Nausea, Vomiting, or Heartburn	
Constipation	+
Diarrhea	
Fatigue	+
Mouth Sores	
Dry Mouth	+
Chewing or Swallowing Difficulty	
Taste Aversion— Sweet	+
Taste Aversion— Sour & Bitter	
Lack of Taste	+
Smells Bother	+

Vegetable Wraps with Edamame Spread ①

Time: 15 minutes
Serves 4

Soybeans are a fun alternative to chickpeas, when it comes to a hummus-like spread. In addition to protein and fiber, soybeans are also a good source of polyunsaturated fats. Enjoy it exactly the same way you would regular hummus.

1½ cups frozen shelled edamame, thawed slightly	½ tablespoon crushed garlic
	½ teaspoon salt
3 tablespoons olive oil	4 whole wheat wraps
½ teaspoon paprika	Sliced cucumber or red bell pepper

1. Warm the edamame in a microwave-safe bowl in the microwave on high power for about 45 seconds, or until the edamame have lost their chill.
2. In a food processor or blender, blend the edamame, olive oil, paprika, crushed garlic, and salt. If it gets too thick, slowly add up to 4 tablespoons of water, 1 tablespoon at a time, until the spread reaches your desired consistency.
3. Smear the edamame spread onto each whole wheat wrap and top with cucumber or red bell pepper slices.

Nutritional Analysis (¼ cup dip + 1 [8-inch] whole wheat wrap): Calories 270, Total Fat 15 g, Saturated Fat 3 g, Cholesterol 0 mg, Sodium 551 mg, Carbohydrates 25 g, Dietary Fiber 5 g, Protein 9 g

---

Sidebar symptoms:

+ Lack of Appetite
+ Nausea, Vomiting, or Heartburn
+ Constipation
+ Diarrhea
+ Fatigue
+ Mouth Sores
+ Dry Mouth
+ Chewing or Swallowing Difficulty
+ Taste Aversion—Sweet
+ Taste Aversion—Sour & Bitter
+ Lack of Taste

Smells Bother

Spiced Lentil Burritos

Time: Prep: 10 minutes; Cook: 30 minutes
Serves 4

A variety of spices are the star of this recipe and pair beautifully with the lentils and leeks. If you are sensitive to spice, consider tabling this recipe for another, less sensitive time. Add shredded chicken, turkey, or tofu, for extra protein.

4 tomatoes, seeded and chopped

1 tablespoon freshly squeezed lime juice

2 tablespoons finely chopped fresh cilantro

2 medium-size leeks, white parts only

1 tablespoon olive oil

¾ teaspoon dried marjoram

¾ teaspoon chili powder

½ teaspoon ground coriander

¼ teaspoon ground cumin

½ teaspoon hot sauce (optional)

2 cups cooked green, black, or brown lentils (if using canned lentils, drain and rinse before using)

4 flour tortillas

½ cup shredded Cheddar or Jack cheese

1. In large bowl, toss the tomatoes, lime juice, and cilantro. Set aside.
2. Cut the leeks in half lengthwise. Clean thoroughly. Chop into small pieces.
3. Heat the olive oil in a large skillet over medium-high heat. Add the leeks, marjoram, chili powder, coriander, cumin, and hot sauce, if using. Sauté until the leeks are tender and translucent, for about 5 minutes. Add the lentils and mix.
4. Divide the mixture into four equal portions and place on the tortillas. Add the cheese and tomato mixture and roll up the tortillas into burritos.

Nutritional Analysis: Calories 451, Total Fat 14 g, Saturated Fat 5 g, Cholesterol 15 mg, Sodium 738 mg, Carbohydrates 66 g, Dietary Fiber 11 g, Protein 20 g

Symptom	
Lack of Appetite	+
Nausea, Vomiting, or Heartburn	
Constipation	+
Diarrhea	
Fatigue	+
Mouth Sores	
Dry Mouth	+
Chewing or Swallowing Difficulty	+
Taste Aversion—Sweet	+
Taste Aversion—Sour & Bitter	
Lack of Taste	+
Smells Bother	

Roasted Vegetable Tostadas

Time: Prep: 15 minutes; Cook: 45 minutes
Serves 2

Who says you have to fry a tostada to make it good? These easy baked tostadas are a great addition to your weeknight dinner routine. To serve, top with shredded lettuce, hot sauce, salsa, sour cream, or avocado. Add some shredded chicken or scrambled eggs, for an extra protein boost.

2 cup cherry or grape tomatoes, halved

1 medium-size red bell pepper, seeded and chopped

1 medium-size white onion, chopped

2 tablespoons olive oil

1 cup black beans (if using canned beans, drain and rinse)

¼ cup chopped fresh cilantro

1 teaspoon garlic powder

4 corn tortillas

½ cup shredded Jack cheese

1. Preheat the oven to 425°F.
2. Toss the tomatoes, pepper, and onion with 1 tablespoon of the olive oil. Place on a baking sheet and roast for 30 minutes.
3. Remove from the oven and toss with the black beans and cilantro. Lower the oven temperature to 375°F.
4. In a small bowl, mix together the remaining tablespoon of olive oil and the garlic powder. Brush the mixture evenly over both sides of the tortillas.
5. Sprinkle the cheese over the tortillas and place one quarter of the bean mixture in the center of each tortilla.
6. Bake for 10 to 15 minutes, until the tortillas are toasted and the cheese has melted. Remove from the oven and cover with the toppings of your choice.

Nutritional Analysis: Calories 496, Total Fat 25 g, Saturated Fat 7 g, Cholesterol 30 mg, Sodium 195 mg, Carbohydrates 53 g, Dietary Fiber 14 g, Protein 19 g

Lack of Appetite

Nausea, Vomiting, or Heartburn

Constipation

Diarrhea

Fatigue

Mouth Sores

Dry Mouth

Chewing or Swallowing Difficulty

Taste Aversion—Sweet

Taste Aversion—Sour & Bitter

Lack of Taste

Smells Bother

Tacos with Peppery Tomato Simmered Lentils

Time: Prep: 15 minutes; Cook: 30 minutes
Serves 4

Lentils are a great source of protein, fiber, and iron, while both lentils and tomatoes give this recipe a nice punch of potassium. For increased calories, add sliced avocado and a dollop of sour cream or plain Greek yogurt to each taco.

1 tablespoon olive oil

1 medium-size yellow onion, chopped

1 medium-size red bell pepper, seeded and chopped

2 garlic cloves, minced

1 (15-ounce) can diced tomatoes in juice

1 cup dried green, black, or brown lentils

1 cup vegetable stock

½ cup fresh cilantro, minced

1 teaspoon chili powder

1 tablespoon honey or agave nectar

1 tablespoon low-sodium soy sauce

½ teaspoon ground cumin

1 bay leaf

8 corn tortillas

2 cups shredded lettuce

½ cup shredded Cheddar cheese

1. Heat the olive oil in a large skillet over medium-high heat. Cook the onion and pepper until shiny and translucent, for 5 to 7 minutes. Add the garlic and cook for another minute.
2. Add the tomatoes, lentils, vegetable stock, cilantro, chili powder, honey, soy sauce, cumin, and bay leaf. Bring to a boil. Lower the heat to low and simmer for 15 to 20 minutes, or until the lentils are cooked and have absorbed most of the stock. Discard the bay leaf.
3. Warm the tortillas in a preheated 350°F oven for 8 to 10 minutes, or heat them over the flame on a gas stove for about 30 seconds. Fill the tortillas with the lentil mixture. Top with the lettuce and cheese.

Nutritional Analysis: Calories 389, Total Fat 10 g, Saturated Fat 3 g, Cholesterol 15 mg, Sodium 500 mg, Carbohydrates 59 g, Dietary Fiber 13 g, Protein 18 g

Symptom	
Lack of Appetite	+
Nausea, Vomiting, or Heartburn	
Constipation	+
Diarrhea	
Fatigue	+
Mouth Sores	
Dry Mouth	+
Chewing or Swallowing Difficulty	+
Taste Aversion— Sweet	
Taste Aversion— Sour & Bitter	
Lack of Taste	+
Smells Bother	

Stretch and Save: Make migas with leftovers. Chop the tortillas into small pieces and sauté on a skillet with a little oil until crunchy. Mix the leftover lentils with a few beaten eggs and add to the skillet with the crunchy tortillas. Cook until the eggs are fully cooked. This is a fun twist on scrambled eggs, with a lentil filling and crunchy yet soft tortilla bites!

Shrimp Salad Sandwiches ◐

Time: Prep: 15 minutes; Cook: 15 minutes
Serves 4

Shrimp are a wonderful low-calorie protein source as well as a good source of iron and omega-3 fatty acids. Cooking them in the shell imparts more flavor than peeling them ahead of time. For a truly decadent sandwich, try it like a lobster roll—serve the shrimp salad in buttered and toasted hot dog buns. Leftovers will keep in the refrigerator for 2 to 3 days.

2 teaspoons salt	1½ teaspoons white wine vinegar
½ lemon, cut into quarters	¼ teaspoon freshly ground black pepper
1 pound large shrimp in the shell (16/20 count)	1½ tablespoons minced fresh dill
	½ small red onion, minced
½ cup mayonnaise or a mix of mayonnaise and plain Greek yogurt	¾ cup minced celery
	2 tablespoons capers
¼ teaspoon Dijon mustard	4 brioche or whole wheat hot dog–style buns, toasted

1. Bring 2½ quarts of water, 1½ teaspoons of the salt, and the lemon to a boil in a large saucepan. Add the shrimp and lower the heat to medium. Cook, uncovered, for 3 minutes, or until the shrimp are just cooked through.
2. Transfer with a slotted spoon to a bowl of ice-cold water.
3. In a separate bowl, whisk together the mayonnaise, mustard, vinegar, remaining ½ teaspoon of salt, pepper, and dill. Combine with the peeled shrimp. Add the red onion, celery, and capers. Serve on top of the toasted brioche.

Nutritional Analysis: Calories 585, Total Fat 32 g, Saturated Fat 8 g, Cholesterol 243 mg, Sodium 1137 mg, Carbohydrates 46 g, Dietary Fiber 4 g, Protein 29 g

Lack of Appetite	+
Nausea, Vomiting, or Heartburn	
Constipation	+
Diarrhea	+
Fatigue	+
Mouth Sores	
Dry Mouth	+
Chewing or Swallowing Difficulty	
Taste Aversion— Sweet	+
Taste Aversion— Sour & Bitter	
Lack of Taste	+
Smells Bother	

Crunchy Tuna Salad Melt

Time: Prep: 30 minutes; Cook: 10 minutes
Serves 6

Lack of Appetite	+
Nausea, Vomiting, or Heartburn	
Constipation	+
Diarrhea	
Fatigue	+
Mouth Sores	
Dry Mouth	+
Chewing or Swallowing Difficulty	+
Taste Aversion— Sweet	
Taste Aversion— Sour & Bitter	
Lack of Taste	+
Smells Bother	

This is not your ordinary tuna salad recipe. Try it in total or pick and choose what sounds good to you at any given time. If you are experiencing nausea and vomiting or sensitive to smells, make a simple tuna sandwich without broiling, as heating the tuna will intensify the fish aroma. Additionally, try a more mild cheese, such as a mild Swiss or Cheddar. The tuna salad can be kept in the refrigerator for 1 to 3 days and can be enjoyed with sliced veggies or crackers as a snack, a healthy wrap with lettuce and tomato, or on a rice cake.

2 (5-ounce) cans tuna in water, drained
1 medium-size red bell pepper, seeded and finely diced
1 medium-size apple, cored and finely diced
1 medium-size carrot, finely diced
½ small red onion, finely diced
1 celery rib, finely diced
½ cup chopped fresh parsley
2 tablespoons Dijon mustard
2 tablespoons plain Greek yogurt
Salt and freshly ground black pepper
6 slices ciabatta bread, halved horizontally
6 slices Swiss cheese

1. Preheat the broiler or preheat the oven to 450°F. Line a baking sheet with parchment paper or foil.
2. In a large bowl, combine the drained tuna, bell pepper, apple, carrot, red onion, celery, and parsley.
3. Add the mustard and Greek yogurt and mix well. Season with salt and black pepper to taste.
4. Place the sliced ciabatta bread, cut side up, on the prepared baking sheet and spoon the tuna salad on top of the ciabatta bottoms.
5. Add a slice of cheese to each ciabatta top and place the baking sheet on the top rack, cheese side up, directly under the broiler. Broil for 1 to 2 minutes or heat in the oven for 4 to 5 minutes, or until the cheese is melted. Watch closely as this will cook quickly.

Nutritional Analysis: Calories 441, Total Fat 10 g, Saturated Fat 5 g, Cholesterol 40 mg, Sodium 775 mg, Carbohydrates 56 g, Dietary Fiber 4 g, Protein 33 g

Nutritionist's Favorite to Savor
This recipe is my favorite because it elevates the clichéd celery and mayo–based tuna salad by jam-packing it with colorful vegetables and fruits. Adding color to meals not only helps make food look more enticing but the varying colors also provide multiple health benefits.

Roasted Eggplant Pesto Sandwich

Time: Prep: 10 minutes; Cook: 30 minutes
Serves 2

Lack of
Appetite

Nausea,
Vomiting, or
Heartburn

Constipation

Diarrhea

Fatigue

Mouth
Sores

Dry
Mouth

Chewing or
Swallowing
Difficulty

Taste
Aversion—
Sweet

Taste
Aversion—
Sour & Bitter

Lack of
Taste

Smells
Bother

This fail-safe roasted eggplant pesto sandwich is sure to become a lunch or dinner staple. Try a splash of balsamic vinegar and fresh basil leaves, for more flavor. Or add some heat with a few sprinkles of red pepper flakes. Creamy hummus or a grilled chicken breast will add protein, if desired.

½ large eggplant, sliced into ¼-inch rounds

1 to 2 tablespoons olive oil

⅛ teaspoon salt

2 rolls ciabatta bread, halved lengthwise

4 tablespoons Basic Pesto (page 219)

4 slices mozzarella cheese

1 avocado, peeled, pitted, and sliced

1. Preheat the oven to 375°F.
2. Coat both sides of the eggplant slices with olive oil and place on a parchment-lined baking sheet. Sprinkle with the salt.
3. Roast the eggplant in the oven for 20 minutes, flipping the slices over halfway through the baking time. Remove the eggplant from the oven, flip again, and cook for another 3 to 5 minutes, or until the slices are moist and slightly browned.
4. Meanwhile, place the ciabatta bread halves on a separate small baking sheet in the oven to toast for about 5 minutes. Take the bread out of the oven, smear with the pesto, place a slice of cheese on each half, and put the bread back in the oven until the cheese is lightly melted.
5. Remove the eggplant and ciabatta from the oven. Once the eggplant is cool enough to handle, prepare the sandwiches by adding the eggplant and avocado slices to the ciabatta.

Nutritional Analysis: Calories 664, Total Fat 50 g, Saturated Fat 12 g, Cholesterol 22 mg, Sodium 777 mg, Carbohydrates 40 g, Dietary Fiber 12 g, Protein 21 g

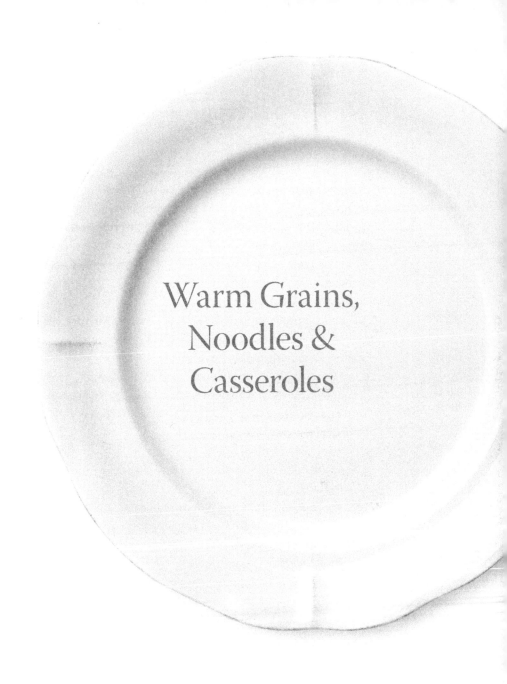

Warm Grains, Noodles & Casseroles

Cheesy Quinoa Poppers with Marinara Dipping Sauce

Time: Prep: 15 minutes; Cook: 30 minutes
Makes 30 bites

+ Lack of Appetite

+ Nausea, Vomiting, or Heartburn

+ Constipation

Diarrhea

+ Fatigue

+ Mouth Sores

+ Dry Mouth

+ Chewing or Swallowing Difficulty

+ Taste Aversion—Sweet

+ Taste Aversion—Sour & Bitter

+ Lack of Taste

+ Smells Bother

These cheesy poppers are so fun to eat! They are like an adult version of chicken nuggets, except they are vegetarian and much better for you. Play around with different herbs and vegetables that you have on hand; just be sure to cut them into small pieces so they cook easily. If you have mouth sores or taste sensitivities, cut down on the spices, garlic, and onion as needed.

Unsalted butter, nonstick cooking spray, or oil, for muffin tin

2 cups cooked quinoa

¼ small red onion, finely chopped

1 cup shredded mozzarella or Gruyère cheese

2 teaspoons minced garlic

½ cup fresh basil, chopped

½ teaspoon salt

1 teaspoon dried oregano

2 large eggs

Mirepoix Marinara Sauce (page 217), for dipping

1. Preheat the oven to 350°F. Grease 30 mini muffin cups with unsalted butter.
2. In a medium-size bowl, mix together the cooked quinoa, red onion, cheese, garlic, basil, salt, oregano, and eggs. Add up to 2 tablespoons of water, 1 tablespoon at a time, as needed, to help the mixture stick together.
3. Distribute the mixture among the prepared mini muffin cups, filling each cup to the top (1 heaping tablespoon each), and press down gently.
4. Bake for 15 to 20 minutes, or until the poppers have browned slightly. Let cool for at least 5 minutes. Use an offset spatula or knife to remove the poppers from the pan.
5. Dip the baked quinoa bites in the marinara sauce.

Nutritional Analysis (per bite): Calories 31, Total Fat 1 g, Saturated Fat 1 g, Cholesterol 16 mg, Sodium 60 mg, Carbohydrates 3 g, Dietary Fiber 0 g, Protein 2 g

Green-Flecked Quinoa Oat Cakes

Time: Prep: 15 minutes; Cook: 30 minutes
Makes 12 cakes

The "green flecks" in these quinoa oat cakes come from nutritious broccoli and fragrant scallions and chopped mint. Lemon zest adds some zing. For added protein and calories, roll the cakes in crushed nuts mixed with some panko crumbs prior to cooking.

1 cup uncooked quinoa, rinsed	¾ cup rolled or quick oats
Salt and freshly ground black pepper	Zest of 1 large or 2 small lemons
1½ cups chopped broccoli florets	½ cup roughly chopped fresh
4 large eggs	mint
6 scallions, chopped	Oil, for cooking

1. Put the quinoa and 2 cups of water in a medium-size pot. Bring to a boil, add a pinch of salt and pepper, lower the heat to a simmer, cover, and cook for 15 minutes. Fluff the quinoa with a fork, turn off the heat, and set the lid ajar for the quinoa to rest.
2. In a food processor, pulse the broccoli until it is reduced to couscous-size pieces, for 10 to 15 pulses.
3. In a large bowl, whisk the eggs well. Add the broccoli to the eggs.
4. Place the scallions and oats in the processor and pulse a few times to roughly chop.
5. Add this to the egg along with the cooked quinoa. Add a generous pinch of salt and pepper and the lemon zest and chopped mint and stir to mix well. Let the mixture rest in the refrigerator for at least 30 minutes.
6. Warm a spoonful of oil in a heavy-bottomed skillet over medium-high heat. Form the quinoa mixture into patties about 4 inches wide and 1 inch thick. Working in batches, cook them for about 4 minutes on each side until just crisped, covering them after they flip to completely warm through. Adding more oil as needed, repeat until all the patties are fried.

Nutritional Analysis (per patty): Calories 121, Total Fat 5 g, Saturated Fat 1 g, Cholesterol 72 mg, Sodium 107 mg, Carbohydrates 14 g, Dietary Fiber 2 g, Protein 5 g

Lack of Appetite	+
Nausea, Vomiting, or Heartburn	+
Constipation	+
Diarrhea	
Fatigue	+
Mouth Sores	+
Dry Mouth	+
Chewing or Swallowing Difficulty	+
Taste Aversion— Sweet	+
Taste Aversion— Sour & Bitter	+
Lack of Taste	+
Smells Bother	+

Warm Quinoa Bowl with Vegetables and Feta

Time: Prep: 15 minutes; Cook: 30 minutes
Serves 6

Lack of
Appetite

Nausea,
Vomiting, or
Heartburn

Constipation

Diarrhea

Fatigue

Mouth
Sores

Dry
Mouth

Chewing or
Swallowing
Difficulty

Taste
Aversion—
Sweet

Taste
Aversion—
Sour & Bitter

Lack of
Taste

Smells
Bother

Cooking the quinoa in vegetable stock adds a lot of flavor. Replace the feta with cannellini beans to make the recipe vegan. This quinoa bowl makes great leftovers that can easily be packed up and eaten anywhere.

3 cups vegetable stock

1½ cups uncooked quinoa, rinsed

1 tablespoon olive oil

3 garlic cloves, minced

1 medium-size yellow onion, diced

3 cups diced zucchini

1 orange bell pepper, seeded and diced

Salt and freshly ground black pepper

2 ounces pasteurized feta or goat cheese, crumbled

2 tablespoons sliced fresh basil leaves

1. Place the vegetable stock in a medium-size saucepan over high heat. Add the quinoa, lower the heat to low, cover, and cook for 15 minutes, or until the liquid has been absorbed. Set aside while you prepare the vegetables.
2. In a large skillet, heat the olive oil over medium heat. Add the garlic and sauté for about a minute. Add the onion, zucchini, and pepper and cook for 7 to 10 minutes, or until the vegetables have started to brown slightly. Season with salt and black pepper to taste.
3. Combine the cooked quinoa with the vegetables. Stir in the cheese (it may start to melt slightly) and basil.

Nutritional Analysis: Calories 235, Total Fat 7 g, Saturated Fat 2 g, Cholesterol 8 mg, Sodium 263 mg, Carbohydrates 35 g, Dietary Fiber 5 g, Protein 9 g

Stretch and Save: Stuff halved peppers, tomatoes, or squash with the leftovers and bake in a preheated 350°F oven until warmed through, for about 30 minutes.

Veggie Paella

Time: Prep: 15 minutes; Cook: 1 hour
Serves 6

Paella is like the Spanish version of risotto, and this dish is sure to please a crowd. Look for tomato paste in a tube rather than a can. Since most recipes only call for a tablespoon or two of tomato paste, squeezing a little from the tube is an easy way to preserve the paste, rather than opening a whole can. The tubes will last in the refrigerator for a long time. Alternatively, if using canned tomato paste, take the remaining paste out of the can and wrap in tightly in a log shape in plastic wrap. Store in the freezer and slice off a little at a time as needed.

½ teaspoon saffron threads

1 tablespoon warm water

2 tablespoons olive oil

1 medium-size onion, chopped

4 garlic cloves, minced

1 medium-size red bell pepper, seeded and cut into strips

1 medium-size yellow bell pepper, seeded and cut into strips

2 cups short-grain brown rice or Arborio rice

1 tablespoon tomato paste

1 teaspoon paprika

1 (15-ounce) can diced tomatoes

4 to 6 cups Aromatic Vegetable Stock (page 216) or water

½ cup chopped fresh or frozen green beans

½ cup chopped canned or frozen baby artichokes

1 (15-ounce) can kidney beans, drained and rinsed

1 cup frozen peas

Salt and freshly ground black pepper

1. Crush the saffron threads and place in a small bowl. Add the warm water; set aside.
2. Heat the oil over medium heat in a large, heavy skillet. Add the onion and cook, stirring, until the onion is tender, for about 5 minutes.
3. Add the garlic and peppers and cook for about 3 minutes more, until the peppers begin to soften.
4. Add the rice, tomato paste, and paprika. Cook, stirring, for 1 minute, or until the grains start to toast and crackle. Add the tomatoes and cook for about 5 minutes more, or until the rice just starts to absorb some of the tomato liquid. Stir in the saffron with its soaking water.

Lack of Appetite	+
Nausea, Vomiting, or Heartburn	
Constipation	+
Diarrhea	+
Fatigue	+
Mouth Sores	
Dry Mouth	+
Chewing or Swallowing Difficulty	+
Taste Aversion— Sweet	+
Taste Aversion— Sour & Bitter	+
Lack of Taste	+
Smells Bother	+

5. Add 2 cups of the stock. Bring to a boil. Stir and then lower the heat to medium-low, and simmer, adding ½ cup more stock at a time every few minutes, until the rice is cooked. This will probably take 30 to 45 minutes more.

6. Add the green beans, artichokes, kidney beans, and peas. Continue to simmer for another 5 to 10 minutes. Remove from the heat and serve with salt and black pepper to taste.

Nutritional Analysis: Calories 409, Total Fat 7 g, Saturated Fat 1 g, Cholesterol 0 mg, Sodium 406 mg, Carbohydrates 79 g, Dietary Fiber 12 g, Protein 11 g

Nutritionist's Favorite to Savor

This recipe is my favorite because it is a plant-based version of an often meat- and seafood-heavy entrée. The recipe fits in peas, artichokes, tomatoes, onions, garlic, and bell peppers for a serious veggie party. Did you know that kidney beans contain more antioxidants than blueberries?!

Harvest Studded Squash

Time: Prep: 30 minutes; Cook: 1 hour
Serves 4

Stuffed squash always looks impressive. Using wild rice instead of brown or white rice adds texture and variety, and more protein and fiber. This dish has a nice sweetness to it from the acorn squash, dried cranberries, and maple syrup.

2 acorn squash, sliced in half and
  seeded
1 tablespoon + 2 teaspoons olive oil
½ cup chopped onion
2 garlic cloves, minced
1 teaspoon dried marjoram
1 tablespoon ground nutmeg
1 cup uncooked wild rice

2 cups Aromatic Vegetable Stock
  (page 216)
2 scallions, chopped
½ cup slivered almonds
½ cup dried cranberries
2 tablespoons pure maple syrup
Juice of ½ orange
Salt and freshly ground pepper

1. Preheat the oven to 400°F. Line a baking sheet with parchment paper. Rub the cut sides of the squash with 2 teaspoons of the olive oil, and place the squash, cut side down, on the prepared baking sheet. Roast for 40 minutes, or until the squash is cooked all the way through.

2. While the squash is cooking, prepare the filling. Heat the remaining tablespoon of olive oil in a large saucepan over medium heat. Add the onion and sauté until soft, for about 5 minutes.

3. Add the garlic and cook for another minute. Add the marjoram, nutmeg, wild rice, and vegetable stock and bring to a boil. Once boiling, lower the heat to a simmer and cook until all the stock has been absorbed. This will take 25 to 40 minutes, depending on the type of wild rice you have. You may need to add more stock or water, as needed, if the rice takes a while to cook.

4. Remove from the heat and fold in the scallions, slivered almonds, cranberries, maple syrup, and orange juice. Season with salt and pepper to taste.

5. Once the acorn squash is finished cooking, stuff with the wild rice mixture.

Lack of Appetite	+
Nausea, Vomiting, or Heartburn	+
Constipation	+
Diarrhea	
Fatigue	+
Mouth Sores	
Dry Mouth	+
Chewing or Swallowing Difficulty	+
Taste Aversion—Sweet	+
Taste Aversion—Sour & Bitter	+
Lack of Taste	+
Smells Bother	+

Nutritional Analysis: Calories 463, Total Fat 14 g, Saturated Fat 2 g, Cholesterol 0 mg, Sodium 204 mg, Carbohydrates 81 g, Dietary Fiber 10 g, Protein 11 g

Paprika Chickpeas over Polenta

Time: Prep: 15 minutes; Cook: 30 minutes
Serves 4

Polenta is basically a cooked cornmeal porridge. Polenta does not have to be made with a package that says "polenta" on it. If you cannot find polenta at your grocery store, you can easily use coarse or medium grind cornmeal. Depending on the type of polenta or cornmeal you use—coarse, medium, or fine grind—it may take anywhere from 15 to 45 minutes to cook. Make this recipe even smoother by replacing chickpeas with softer cannellini beans; reduce the tomatoes as needed to tone down the acidity.

2 cups cherry or grape tomatoes

1 tablespoon + 1 teaspoon olive oil

½ medium-size yellow onion, diced

1½ cups cooked chickpeas, or
   1 (15-ounce) can, drained and rinsed

1 teaspoon paprika or smoked paprika

1 cup polenta

½ cup grated Parmesan cheese

Salt and freshly ground black pepper

Greek yogurt, for serving

1. Preheat the oven to 400°F.
2. Roast the tomatoes: Toss the tomatoes with 1 teaspoon of the olive oil and roast in the oven until soft but not totally shapeless, for 15 to 20 minutes. Remove from the heat and set aside.
3. Heat the remaining tablespoon of olive oil in a skillet over medium-high heat and sauté the onion until slightly softened, for about 5 minutes. Add the chickpeas and paprika, and continue to sauté for another 2 to 3 minutes. Remove from the heat and set aside.
4. Prepare the polenta: Place 4 cups of water in a pot along with the polenta. Bring to a low simmer, stirring frequently so the polenta does not burn. When the water has absorbed and the polenta is cooked (it may take anywhere from 15 to 45 minutes to cook), turn off the heat.
5. Add the Parmesan cheese, a generous quantity of pepper, and a pinch of salt.
6. Divide the polenta among four bowls. To each bowl, add a dollop of Greek yogurt, a large spoonful of the chickpeas, and one quarter of the cherry tomatoes. Serve warm.

Lack of Appetite	+
Nausea, Vomiting, or Heartburn	
Constipation	
Diarrhea	+
Fatigue	+
Mouth Sores	
Dry Mouth	+
Chewing or Swallowing Difficulty	+
Taste Aversion— Sweet	+
Taste Aversion— Sour & Bitter	+
Lack of Taste	+
Smells Bother	+

Nutritional Analysis (not including Greek yogurt): Calories 351, Total Fat 9 g, Saturated Fat 3 g, Cholesterol 9 mg, Sodium 433 mg, Carbohydrates 55 g, Dietary Fiber 5 g, Protein 13 g

Stretch and Save: Turn leftovers into a "polenta pizza." Spread a thin layer of leftover polenta over the bottom of a baking sheet. Heat in a preheated 400°F oven with the tomatoes and some extra cheese for 10 to 15 minutes. Cut into strips and eat it like a pizza.

Udon Noodles with Sesame Soy Snap Peas

Time: Prep: 15 minutes; Cook: 30 minutes
Serves 2

Don't have udon noodles? Try this with soba noodles, whole wheat spaghetti, or zucchini noodles. Toss in cooked tofu, chicken, beef, or shrimp to get a boost of extra protein. Substitute cooked snow peas for sugar snap peas if chewing is an issue. Or eat the noodles by themselves with the sauce for a simple, comforting dish.

10 ounces sugar snap peas

1 tablespoon olive oil

Pinch of salt

4 ounces udon noodles

For the dressing

1 tablespoon low-sodium soy sauce

1 tablespoon brown rice vinegar

2 teaspoons sesame oil

1 tablespoon honey

2 tablespoons toasted sesame seeds

1 teaspoon minced fresh ginger (optional)

1. Preheat the oven to 375°F.
2. Rinse the snap peas, toss with the olive oil and salt, and spread out on a baking sheet. Roast until tender and brown spots begin to develop, for 15 to 20 minutes.
3. While roasting the snap peas, prepare the udon noodles according to the package directions.
4. Make the dressing: Whisk together the soy sauce, vinegar, sesame oil, honey, 1 tablespoon of the sesame seeds, and the ginger, if using. Taste and adjust the flavoring as needed.
5. To serve, toss the noodles, snap peas, and dressing together. Sprinkle with the remaining tablespoon of sesame seeds.

Nutritional Analysis: Calories 458, Total Fat 17 g, Saturated Fat 2 g, Cholesterol 0 mg, Sodium 381 mg, Carbohydrates 62 g, Dietary Fiber 8 g, Protein 14 g

Symptom	
Lack of Appetite	+
Nausea, Vomiting, or Heartburn	
Constipation	+
Diarrhea	
Fatigue	+
Mouth Sores	+
Dry Mouth	+
Chewing or Swallowing Difficulty	+
Taste Aversion— Sweet	+
Taste Aversion— Sour & Bitter	+
Lack of Taste	+
Smells Bother	

Your Way Zucchini Noodles ◑

Time: Prep: 10 minutes; Cook: 15 minutes
Serves 4

Lack of
Appetite

Nausea,
Vomiting, or
Heartburn

Constipation

Diarrhea

Fatigue

Mouth
Sores

Dry
Mouth

Chewing or
Swallowing
Difficulty

Taste
Aversion—
Sweet

Taste
Aversion—
Sour & Bitter

Lack of
Taste

Smells
Bother

Keep the noodles raw for extra crunch, or blanch them in boiling water for 30 seconds to add a little tenderness, then place in an ice bath to prevent overcooking. Drain from the ice bath and toss with your favorite sauce. Zucchini is a very mild vegetable that is versatile for many symptoms because it is easy to digest.

4 medium-size zucchini

1 cup cherry or grape tomatoes, halved

Mediterranean Artichoke Olive Sauce (page 221), Kale Pesto (page 218), or Mirepoix Marinara Sauce (page 217)

1. Rinse the zucchini well, pat dry, and chop the ends off.
2. Using a spiralizer or julienne peeler, make noodles out of all the zucchini and place in a large serving bowl. Note: Once you get to the last 2 inches or so of the zucchini, it will be difficult to spiralize or peel, so you can either grate it or finely chop the rest.
3. Add the cherry tomatoes and top with the sauce of your choice.

Nutritional Analysis (not including sauce): Calories 40, Total Fat 1 g, Saturated Fat 0 g, Cholesterol 0 mg, Sodium 18 mg, Carbohydrates 8 g, Dietary Fiber 2 g, Protein 3 g

Sweet Potato and Broccoli Mac and Cheese

Time: Prep: 30 minutes; Cook: 45 minutes
Serves 6

This baked mac and cheese has all the gooey goodness of traditional mac, but with extra nutrition from using whole wheat noodles and adding mashed sweet potato and broccoli. Steam the broccoli before adding it to the mac for extra tenderness and ease in chewing and swallowing.

1 medium-size sweet potato

1½ cups milk

3 cups dried whole wheat pasta

¾ cup shredded mozzarella cheese

¾ cup shredded Asiago cheese

½ cup shredded Parmesan cheese

2 tablespoons unsalted butter

2 garlic cloves, minced

2 tablespoons all-purpose flour

2 heaping cups fresh or frozen broccoli,
    cut into small pieces

1. Preheat the oven to 400°F.
2. Peel and cube the sweet potato. Bring a pot of water to a boil, add the sweet potato, and cook until tender, for 8 to 12 minutes.
3. Drain and let cool slightly. Place the cooked sweet potato in a food processor with ¼ cup of the milk. Pulse until smooth and set aside.
4. Bring a fresh pot of water to a boil and cook the pasta for 5 to 6 minutes. The pasta should still be al dente. Drain and set aside.
5. Mix the cheeses together and set aside.
6. In a saucepan, melt the butter, add the garlic, and cook for 1 minute. Whisk in the flour and let cook for another 1 to 2 minutes, whisking constantly, to cook out the flour taste.
7. Whisk in the remaining 1¼ cups of milk and cook, stirring constantly, until the mixture begins to thicken.
8. Whisk in the sweet potato puree and continue to cook until hot, stirring often to prevent burning. Remove from the heat and add 1½ cups of the cheese mixture.
9. In a large casserole dish, stir together the pasta, broccoli, and cheese sauce. Toss until the broccoli begins to brighten and the cheese is melting in.
10. Sprinkle the remaining cheese on top. Bake for 25 to 35 minutes, or until the cheese on top starts to brown all over.

Symptom	
Lack of Appetite	+
Nausea, Vomiting, or Heartburn	+
Constipation	+
Diarrhea	
Fatigue	+
Mouth Sores	+
Dry Mouth	+
Chewing or Swallowing Difficulty	+
Taste Aversion—Sweet	+
Taste Aversion—Sour & Bitter	+
Lack of Taste	+
Smells Bother	+

Nutritional Analysis: Calories 401, Total Fat 15 g, Saturated Fat 8 g, Cholesterol 38 mg, Sodium 383 mg, Carbohydrates 52 g, Dietary Fiber 6 g, Protein 21 g

Creamy Grits with Roasted Tomatoes and Sautéed Spinach

Time: Prep: 15 minutes; Cook: 30 minutes
Serves 3

Not only do grits taste good, they also cook up in just 5 minutes! For a variation on the spinach, swap in some stronger tasting yet highly nutritious mustard greens or broccoli rabe. If you need extra protein, top with sautéed shrimp for the classic shrimp and grits combo. If experiencing nausea, a bowl of plain grits with a small amount of butter and a pinch of salt can be a warm, comforting dish.

1 cup cherry or grape tomatoes, halved	½ cup shredded Cheddar cheese
1 tablespoon + 1 teaspoon olive oil	Dash of hot sauce (optional)
1 cup milk	1 garlic clove, minced
½ teaspoon salt	½ cup vegetable stock
¾ cup uncooked grits	3 cups chopped spinach

1. Preheat the oven to 425°F.
2. Place the tomatoes on a baking sheet and drizzle with the teaspoon of olive oil. Bake until the skins shimmer and begin to burst, for 15 to 20 minutes. Remove from the oven and set aside.
3. Bring the milk, 2 cups of water, and the salt to a boil in a medium-size saucepan on medium-high heat. Slowly add the grits, stirring constantly to prevent lumps from forming. Lower the heat to medium-low and cook for 5 minutes, stirring occasionally. Once cooked, remove from the heat and stir in the cheese and hot sauce, if using. Cover and set aside. The grits will thicken slightly as they cool.
4. Meanwhile, heat the remaining tablespoon of olive oil in a large skillet over medium-high heat. Add the garlic and sauté for 1 minute. Add the vegetable stock and spinach and sauté until the greens are wilted and the stock has mostly evaporated.
5. Plate the grits in serving bowls, then add a generous serving of spinach, followed by the roasted tomatoes. Dot with hot sauce, if using.

Lack of Appetite	+
Nausea, Vomiting, or Heartburn	+
Constipation	+
Diarrhea	
Fatigue	+
Mouth Sores	
Dry Mouth	+
Chewing or Swallowing Difficulty	+
Taste Aversion— Sweet	+
Taste Aversion— Sour & Bitter	+
Lack of Taste	+
Smells Bother	+

Nutritional Analysis: Calories 333, Total Fat 13 g, Saturated Fat 5 g, Cholesterol 24 mg, Sodium 540 mg, Carbohydrates 43 g, Dietary Fiber 3 g, Protein 11 g

Stretch and Save: Turn leftovers into mini grits cakes. Spread leftovers into the bottom of a greased loaf pan or 8 by 8-inch baking dish. Cover and refrigerate overnight. The grits will harden slightly. The next day, cut the hardened grits cakes into squares or wedges and sauté in a skillet until slightly toasted and heated through.

Fettuccine with Green Alfredo

Time: Prep: 15 minutes; Cook: 30 minutes
Serves 4

The classic fettuccine Alfredo dish is loaded with calories and saturated fat. This recipe still has a richness to it, but most of the fat is monounsaturated, healthy fat from the avocados. Make this a complete meal by adding protein-rich seared tofu or chicken. Want an even greener flavor? Toss ½ cup of fresh basil into the avocado puree.

10 to 12 small tomatoes

3 tablespoons olive oil

8 ounces fettuccine pasta

2 medium-size avocados, peeled and pitted

2 garlic cloves, roughly chopped

½ teaspoon salt

2 tablespoons freshly squeezed lemon juice

¼ cup grated fresh Pecorino or Parmesan cheese (optional)

¼ cup almond slivers (optional)

Salt and freshly ground black pepper

1. Preheat the oven to 300°F.
2. Wash and quarter the tomatoes. Place on a baking sheet lined with parchment paper. Drizzle with 1 tablespoon of the olive oil, just enough to make the tomatoes glisten. Bake for 20 minutes.
3. Meanwhile, cook the fettuccine according to the package directions.
4. While the pasta is boiling, place the remaining 2 tablespoons of olive oil and the avocado, garlic, salt, and lemon juice in a food processor. Pulse until the sauce is smooth and creamy.
5. Drain the pasta. Combine with the sauce in a large bowl, until all the pasta has been covered.
6. Add the roasted tomatoes and sprinkle with cheese and almond slivers, if using. Add extra salt and pepper to taste.

Nutritional Analysis (without optional toppings): Calories 501, Total Fat 26 g, Saturated Fat 4 g, Cholesterol 0 mg, Sodium 262 mg, Carbohydrates 61 g, Dietary Fiber 11 g, Protein 12 g

Lack of Appetite	+
Nausea, Vomiting, or Heartburn	+
Constipation	+
Diarrhea	
Fatigue	+
Mouth Sores	
Dry Mouth	+
Chewing or Swallowing Difficulty	+
Taste Aversion— Sweet	+
Taste Aversion— Sour & Bitter	+
Lack of Taste	+
Smells Bother	+

Nutritional Analysis (includes 1 tablespoon grated Parmesan and 1 tablespoon slivered almonds): Calories 561, Total Fat 30 g, Saturated Fat 5 g, Cholesterol 4 mg, Sodium 352 mg, Carbohydrates 63 g, Dietary Fiber 12 g, Protein 14 g

Seitan Marinara Pasta Casserole

Time: Prep: 15 minutes; Cook: 1 hour
Serves 8

Seitan mimics the taste and mouthfeel of common animal proteins and it adds a savory element to this pasta casserole. It can be helpful to have your freezer stocked with healthy homemade meals for those times when you don't feel like cooking. Casseroles are great for freezing. To freeze this casserole, cut into individual portions and freeze in resealable plastic bags or airtight containers.

1 (8-ounce) package seitan
2 tablespoons olive oil
1 medium-size onion, chopped
1 medium-size orange or yellow bell pepper, seeded and chopped
¼ cup finely diced broccoli
¼ cup finely diced carrots

1 cup sliced mushrooms
1 (15-ounce) can diced tomatoes
2 cups marinara sauce
1 teaspoon salt
½ teaspoon Italian seasoning
8 ounces whole wheat elbow macaroni
8 ounces shredded mozzarella cheese

1. Chop the seitan into very small pieces.
2. Heat 1 tablespoon of the olive oil in a large, deep skillet over medium-high heat, add the seitan, and cook until browned, for about 5 minutes. Transfer to a plate and set aside. Preheat the oven to 350°F.
3. Place the remaining tablespoon of olive oil in the skillet over medium heat and add the onion, bell pepper, broccoli, carrots, and mushrooms. Sauté until the vegetables soften, for 6 to 7 minutes.
4. Return the seitan to the skillet along with the diced tomatoes, marinara sauce, 1 cup of water, and the salt and Italian seasoning.
5. Bring to a boil, lower the heat to medium-low, and simmer for 5 minutes.
6. Spoon just enough of the seitan and vegetable mixture to cover the bottom of a 9 by 13-inch pan. Cover with the uncooked pasta. Spoon the remaining sauce mixture evenly over the top and sprinkle with the cheese.
7. Cover the pan with foil and bake for 50 to 55 minutes. Remove from the oven and let stand, covered, for 15 minutes. Serve.

Lack of Appetite	+
Nausea, Vomiting, or Heartburn	
Constipation	+
Diarrhea	+
Fatigue	+
Mouth Sores	
Dry Mouth	+
Chewing or Swallowing Difficulty	+
Taste Aversion— Sweet	+
Taste Aversion— Sour & Bitter	+
Lack of Taste	+
Smells Bother	+

Nutritional Analysis: Calories 307, Total Fat 11 g, Saturated Fat 4 g, Cholesterol 15 mg, Sodium 706 mg, Carbohydrates 36 g, Dietary Fiber 4 g, Protein 22 g

Linguine Presto with Tomatoes, Basil, and Garlic ⓘ

Time: Prep: 15 minutes; Cook: 15 minutes
Serves 6

This pasta dish is super easy to prepare—that's why it is called "presto"! The pasta and the sauce cook simultaneously in one pot, and you don't even have to drain the pasta. Toss in some white beans if you desire more protein.

....

12 ounces whole wheat or spinach
    linguine

2 cups cherry or grape tomatoes,
    halved or quartered if large

1 medium-size onion, thinly sliced

6 garlic cloves, thinly sliced

¼ teaspoon red pepper flakes (optional)

2 sprigs basil, plus extra torn leaves,
    for garnish

2 tablespoons olive oil

2 teaspoons salt

¼ teaspoon freshly ground black pepper

Pecorino Romano or Parmesan cheese,
    for serving

....

1. Combine the pasta, tomatoes, onion, garlic, red pepper flakes, basil, oil, salt, black pepper, and 4½ cups of water in a large pot. Bring to a boil over high heat.

2. Boil the mixture, stirring and turning pasta frequently with tongs, until the pasta is al dente and the water has nearly evaporated, about 9 minutes.

3. Divide among four bowls, and garnish with the extra basil. Serve with grated cheese.

Nutritional Analysis: Calories 258, Total Fat 5 g, Saturated Fat 1 g, Cholesterol 0 mg, Sodium 648 mg, Carbohydrates 47 g, Dietary Fiber 8 g, Protein 9 g

Lack of Appetite	+
Nausea, Vomiting, or Heartburn	
Constipation	+
Diarrhea	
Fatigue	+
Mouth Sores	+
Dry Mouth	+
Chewing or Swallowing Difficulty	+
Taste Aversion— Sweet	+
Taste Aversion— Sour & Bitter	+
Lack of Taste	+
Smells Bother	+

Whole Wheat Couscous Primavera

Time: Prep: 15 minutes; Cook: 30 minutes
Serves 8

Lack of
Appetite

Nausea,
Vomiting, or
Heartburn

Constipation

Diarrhea

Fatigue

Mouth
Sores

Dry
Mouth

Chewing or
Swallowing
Difficulty

Taste
Aversion—
Sweet

Taste
Aversion—
Sour & Bitter

Lack of
Taste

Smells
Bother

Couscous is a quick-cooking grain, and using whole wheat couscous adds extra whole-grain nutrients, such as fiber and B vitamins. This primavera is loaded with colorful vegetables and pesto. Serve leftover couscous mixed with a side of Lemony Chickpeas with Parsley (page 81) or alongside some Baked Parmesan Swiss Chard Chips (page 164).

1 cup uncooked whole wheat couscous	1 cup cherry or grape tomatoes, halved
1 tablespoon olive oil	1 teaspoon minced garlic (optional)
½ cup chopped fresh or frozen broccoli	¼ cup Basic Pesto (page 219)
½ cup chopped cauliflower	¼ cup grated Parmesan cheese
½ cup chopped carrots	1 tablespoon freshly squeezed
½ cup chopped cremini mushrooms	lemon juice
½ cup chopped zucchini	Fresh basil, cut into ribbons

1. Cook the couscous according to the package directions.
2. In a large skillet, heat the olive oil over medium-high heat. Add the broccoli, cauliflower, and carrots. Sauté for about 5 minutes. Add the mushrooms and zucchini and sauté for another 5 minutes. You may need to add a splash of water and cover the pan to cook the vegetables more thoroughly. Add the tomatoes and garlic, if using, and sauté for another minute.
3. Add the cooked couscous, pesto, half of the cheese, and the lemon juice. Toss in the pan until well combined. Remove from the heat and add the basil. Sprinkle with the remaining cheese before serving.

Nutritional Analysis: Calories 146, Total Fat 6 g, Saturated Fat 1 g, Cholesterol 3 mg, Sodium 82 mg, Carbohydrates 20 g, Dietary Fiber 4 g, Protein 5 g

Broccoli Kale Lasagne

Time: Prep: 30 minutes; Cook: 1 hour
Serves 8

The layered look is in, and this veggie-centric lasagne is spot on. Use whole milk ricotta cheese if you are trying to get in extra calories, or use Tofu Ricotta (page 225), for a vegan option. The whole family will love this recipe. Want to make the meal extra special? Serve the lasagne with homemade garlic bread. Drizzle olive oil over sliced bread, add garlic powder and/or chopped garlic, a pinch of salt, a sprinkle of Parmesan cheese, and lots of chopped fresh parsley. Bake in a preheated 375°F oven for 10 to 15 minutes.

1 tablespoon olive oil, plus more for baking pan

½ medium-size onion, chopped

2 tablespoons minced garlic

3 cups chopped broccoli, mushrooms, and red or orange bell peppers

½ teaspoon salt

1 large egg

2 cup part-skim ricotta cheese or Tofu Ricotta (page 225)

2 cups chopped fresh kale

3 cups tomato sauce

12 uncooked oven-ready whole wheat lasagna noodles

1 cup shredded mozzarella cheese

1. Preheat the oven to 375°F. Grease a 9 by 13-inch baking pan with olive oil.
2. Heat the 1 tablespoon of olive oil in a large skillet over medium-high heat. Sauté the onion and garlic in the oil. Add the veggies and sauté until tender, for 5 to 8 minutes more. Set aside.
3. Whisk the salt and the egg into ricotta cheese and stir in the chopped kale.
4. Pour about ½ cup of the tomato sauce in the bottom of the prepared baking pan.
5. Top with four lasagna noodles, ½ cup of the ricotta mixture, half of the veggies, and ¾ cup of sauce. Repeat for another layer. Top the pan with the remaining noodles, remaining sauce, and mozzarella cheese.
6. Cover tightly with foil and bake for 40 minutes. Remove the foil and bake for 10 minutes more, or until the cheese is bubbly.

Symptom	
Lack of Appetite	+
Nausea, Vomiting, or Heartburn	
Constipation	+
Diarrhea	
Fatigue	+
Mouth Sores	
Dry Mouth	+
Chewing or Swallowing Difficulty	+
Taste Aversion—Sweet	+
Taste Aversion—Sour & Bitter	+
Lack of Taste	+
Smells Bother	+

Nutritional Analysis: Calories 328, Total Fat 12 g, Saturated Fat 5 g, Cholesterol 54 mg, Sodium 790 mg, Carbohydrates 38 g, Dietary Fiber 8 g, Protein 21 g

Spinach and Scallion Enchiladas

Time: Prep: 15 minutes; Cook: 30 minutes
Serves 4

These skillet enchiladas are quick and easy. Vegetables get sautéed and stuffed into tortillas with some cheese. The rolled tortillas then get added back to the skillet, covered with salsa, and simmered until warmed through. Add chopped tofu or cooked chicken to the filling to up the protein. For a larger meal, spoon the filling into a large flour tortilla and eat as a burrito.

2 tablespoons olive oil
2 cups chopped spinach
½ cup minced scallions
8 corn tortillas

1 cup shredded white Cheddar or Jack cheese
1 cup Tomato Habanero Salsa (page 212)
½ cup plain yogurt

1. In large skillet over medium-high heat, heat 1 tablespoon of the olive oil and sauté the spinach and scallions until the spinach is wilted and the scallions are translucent. Remove from the heat.
2. Divide the mixture equally among the eight tortillas. Top with the cheese. Roll up the tortillas.
3. Place the remaining tablespoon of olive oil in a large skillet over medium heat. Add the rolled tortillas and brown for about 5 minutes on each side. Add the salsa on top. Cover the skillet, lower the heat to medium-low, and simmer for 5 minutes. Remove from the heat, transfer to a plate, and scoop yogurt on top.

Nutritional Analysis: Calories 294, Total Fat 17 g, Saturated Fat 6 g, Cholesterol 32 mg, Sodium 367 mg, Carbohydrates 52 g, Dietary Fiber 4 g, Protein 12 g

Symptom	
Lack of Appetite	+
Nausea, Vomiting, or Heartburn	
Constipation	+
Diarrhea	
Fatigue	+
Mouth Sores	
Dry Mouth	+
Chewing or Swallowing Difficulty	+
Taste Aversion—Sweet	+
Taste Aversion—Sour & Bitter	+
Lack of Taste	+
Smells Bother	+

Walnut-Crusted Spinach and Feta Pie

Time: Prep: 15 minutes; Cook: 30 minutes
Serves 6

This is a great holiday recipe reminiscent of a spinach soufflé with a thin bottom layer of crust. It can be served for breakfast, brunch, lunch, or dinner. You may also substitute ricotta for the feta cheese, for a milder flavor. The cinnamon gives this dish a distinct Mediterranean feel. Mixing ground walnuts with panko provides healthy omega-3 fats and some protein, too.

1 pound fresh or frozen spinach

6 large eggs

½ cup plain yogurt

¼ cup pasteurized feta or goat cheese, crumbled

2 garlic cloves, minced

1 teaspoon dried oregano

½ teaspoon ground cinnamon

¼ cup panko or bread crumbs

3 tablespoons ground walnuts

½ teaspoon olive oil

1. Preheat the oven to 400°F.
2. Place the spinach in large pot with ¼ cup of water. Cook over medium heat until wilted and most of the water is evaporated. Remove from the heat, let cool, and squeeze the remaining liquid from the leaves. Transfer to a food processor and chop into small pieces. Transfer to a large bowl.
3. Add the eggs, yogurt, cheese, garlic, oregano, and cinnamon and stir to combine.
4. In a small bowl, combine the panko and chopped walnuts. Coat a 9-inch pie plate or baking dish with the olive oil. Press the walnut mixture into an even layer on the bottom of the pan.
5. Pour the spinach mixture evenly over the walnut crust. Bake for 30 to 40 minutes.

Nutritional Analysis: Calories 163, Total Fat 9 g, Saturated Fat 3 g, Cholesterol 222 mg, Sodium 211 mg, Carbohydrates 9 g, Dietary Fiber 3 g, Protein 12 g

+	Lack of Appetite
+	Nausea, Vomiting, or Heartburn
+	Constipation
	Diarrhea
+	Fatigue
+	Mouth Sores
+	Dry Mouth
+	Chewing or Swallowing Difficulty
+	Taste Aversion—Sweet
+	Taste Aversion—Sour & Bitter
+	Lack of Taste
+	Smells Bother

Tasty Tofu, Quinoa, and Asparagus Casserole

Time: Prep: 15 minutes; Cook: 30 minutes
Serves 6

 Whenever you see asparagus at your farmers' market, that means spring has arrived! Since the recipe contains quinoa, tofu, and asparagus, it is a complete nutritious meal all baked into one delicious dish. This casserole can easily be customized for your taste. Try swapping out the paprika and dried basil for other spices of preference, such as turmeric and fresh thyme. Instead of quinoa, try the recipe with another quick-cooking grain, such as bulgur wheat or couscous.

Unsalted butter, nonstick cooking spray, or oil, for baking dish	1 (14-ounce) package firm tofu
2 cups vegetable stock	½ teaspoon paprika
1 cup milk	½ teaspoon dried basil
½ cup all-purpose flour	½ teaspoon salt
1 cup uncooked quinoa, rinsed	3 cups chopped asparagus
	¼ cup shredded Gruyère cheese

1. Preheat the oven to 400°F and generously grease a 9 by 13-inch baking dish with unsalted butter.
2. Heat the vegetable stock and milk in a saucepan over medium heat and bring to a low boil. Slowly whisk in the flour, whisking continuously until it thickens into a smooth, creamy sauce. Turn off the heat.
3. Transfer the sauce to a large bowl, add 1 cup of water and the quinoa, and stir to combine. Pour the mixture into the prepared baking dish.
4. Slice the tofu into thin strips and lay the tofu strips over the top of the quinoa mixture. Sprinkle with the paprika, basil, and salt. Bake, uncovered, for 30 minutes.
5. Meanwhile, blanch the asparagus in boiling water for 30 seconds until it turns bright green. Immediately transfer to a bowl filled with ice water. Set aside.
6. Remove the casserole from the oven, check the mixture by stirring it around in the pan, and, if needed, bake for an additional 10 to 15 minutes, until the quinoa is cooked.

Lack of Appetite	+
Nausea, Vomiting, or Heartburn	+
Constipation	+
Diarrhea	+
Fatigue	+
Mouth Sores	+
Dry Mouth	+
Chewing or Swallowing Difficulty	+
Taste Aversion—Sweet	+
Taste Aversion—Sour & Bitter	+
Lack of Taste	+
Smells Bother	+

7. Drain the blanched asparagus from the ice water bath and add it to the casserole with up to 1 cup of water, until the consistency is creamy and smooth and you can stir it easily in the pan.
8. Top with the cheese and bake for 5 more minutes, or just long enough to melt the cheese.

Nutritional Analysis: Calories 252, Total Fat 7 g, Saturated Fat 2 g, Cholesterol 7 mg, Sodium 245 mg, Carbohydrates 33 g, Dietary Fiber 5 g, Protein 15 g

Nutritionist's Favorite to Savor
This recipe is my favorite because asparagus contains a compound called glutathione that may help the body break down carcinogens and other harmful compounds known as free radicals. Glutathione can also be found in such foods as avocado, kale, and Brussels sprouts.

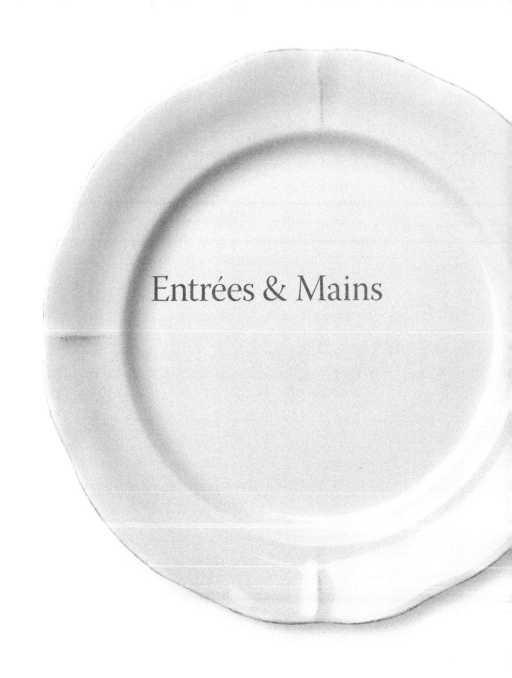

Entrées & Mains

Cheesy Lentil "Meatballs"

Time: Prep: 15 minutes; Cook: 30 minutes
Serves 6

A perfect mini meal for those consuming small, frequent meals to manage digestive symptoms. Try them by themselves or in a pita with our Super-smooth Ginger Hummus (page 223) and creamy Cucumber Tzatziki (page 215). Alternatively, omit the cumin and dip the meatballs in our Mirepoix Marinara Sauce (page 217)! Reduce or omit the cumin as needed if sensitive to the spice. Freeze leftover meatballs in resealable plastic bags or airtight containers for up to a month.

1½ cups cooked or 1 (15-ounce) can green or brown lentils, drained and rinsed if using canned

¾ cup cottage cheese

2 large eggs, lightly beaten

¼ cup grated Parmesan cheese

1 large garlic clove, minced

½ teaspoon ground cumin

2 tablespoons finely chopped fresh cilantro

Hefty pinch of dried or fresh thyme

1 teaspoon salt

¼ teaspoon freshly ground black pepper

⅔ cup panko or bread crumbs, plus more if needed

Olive oil, for brushing (optional)

1. In a food processor, pulverize the lentils and cottage cheese into mush. Transfer to a large bowl.
2. Add the beaten eggs, Parmesan, garlic, cumin, cilantro, thyme, salt, and pepper to the lentil mixture and stir to mix well.
3. Stir in the panko and let the mixture sit for 20 minutes. Meanwhile, preheat the oven to 400°F. Line a baking sheet with parchment paper.
4. Check the lentil mixture by rolling a 1-inch ball between your palms. It should be sticky and wet but hold together fairly well. If it seems too wet and it is falling apart, stir in another 1 to 2 tablespoons of panko, until a ball stays together. Roll the mixture into balls and line them up on the prepared baking sheet. If you like a bit more of a crust, brush them with olive oil.
5. Bake on the middle rack for 15 to 20 minutes, gently turning the balls over halfway through baking, until the tops are golden brown.
6. Remove from the oven and let cool slightly. Serve.

Lack of Appetite

Nausea, Vomiting, or Heartburn

Constipation

Diarrhea

Fatigue

Mouth Sores

Dry Mouth

Chewing or Swallowing Difficulty

Taste Aversion— Sweet

Taste Aversion— Sour & Bitter

Lack of Taste

Smells Bother

Nutritional Analysis: Calories 155, Total Fat 4 g, Saturated Fat 1 g, Cholesterol 76 mg, Sodium 523 mg, Carbohydrates 18 g, Dietary Fiber 4 g, Protein 12 g

Nutritionist's Favorite to Savor
This recipe is my favorite because it contains good protein from the lentils and cottage cheese and a hint of cumin, and the meatballs still have the same look and feel of traditional meat-based meatballs. Try them with spaghetti and red sauce, stuffed into a pita, or smashed onto an egg sandwich.

Eggplant and Kidney Bean "Meatballs" ◐

Time: Prep: 15 minutes; Cook: 15 minutes
Serves 4

This is a great recipe to make in multiple batches and freeze extras for another day. Serve them with pesto instead of marinara and enjoy atop a salad. Or try them over a bed of cooked creamy polenta or farro for an alternative to pasta.

Nonstick cooking spray

1 tablespoon olive oil

1 medium-size unpeeled eggplant, cut into 1-inch pieces

1 teaspoon salt

½ teaspoon freshly ground black pepper

1 medium-size onion, chopped

1 tablespoon minced garlic

1 cup cooked kidney beans (if using canned beans, drain and rinse)

¼ cup chopped fresh parsley

1 cup panko or bread crumbs

Pinch of red pepper flakes (optional)

2 cups marinara sauce or Mirepoix Marinara Sauce (page 217)

1. Preheat the oven to 375°F. Spray a large, rimmed baking sheet with cooking spray.
2. Heat ½ tablespoon of the olive oil in a large, nonstick skillet over medium-high heat. When hot, add the eggplant and ¼ cup of water. Season with salt and pepper and cook, stirring occasionally, until tender, for 10 to 15 minutes. Transfer the eggplant to the bowl of a food processor.
3. Heat the remaining ½ tablespoon of olive oil in the skillet, add the onion and garlic, and cook until translucent, for 3 to 5 minutes.
4. Add to the food processor along with the beans and parsley and pulse until well combined and chopped. Do not puree.
5. Combine the mixture with the panko and red pepper flakes, if using. Roll into twelve meatballs about 2 inches in diameter. Transfer to the prepared baking sheet and bake until firm and browned, for 25 to 30 minutes.
6. Meanwhile, warm the marinara sauce and serve with the meatballs over pasta, zucchini noodles, or smashed onto a whole wheat sub roll.

Nutritional Analysis (not including marinara sauce): Calories 199, Total Fat 4 g, Saturated Fat 1 g, Cholesterol 0 mg, Sodium 601 mg, Carbohydrates 35 g, Dietary Fiber 8 g, Protein 7 g

Vegetarian Sausage

Time: Prep: 15 minutes; Cook: 30 minutes
Serves 4

Try these savory vegetarian sausages any time of the day. Perfect by themselves as a snack for someone trying to eat small, frequent meals; with a side of scrambled eggs or any of our breakfast hashes; or atop a salad for lunch. Leftovers can be refrigerated for up to 5 days or frozen for up to a month.

½ medium-size onion, minced

3 tablespoons olive oil

1 cup minced dinosaur (lacinato) kale

2 tablespoons grated Pecorino Romano or Parmesan cheese

3 garlic cloves, minced

2 cups cold cooked brown rice

1 cup cooked kidney beans (if using canned beans, drain and rinse)

1 large egg white

1 teaspoon finely minced fresh thyme

1 teaspoon finely minced fresh oregano

1 teaspoon finely minced fresh sage

½ cup panko or bread crumbs

1. In a large skillet over medium-high heat, sauté the onion in 1 tablespoon of the olive oil until translucent, for about 5 minutes. Add the kale, cheese, and garlic. Sauté until the kale is wilted, for about 3 minutes more. Remove excess moisture from the mixture by placing it on a double layer of paper towels and patting the top of the mixture with paper towels until the majority of the moisture is removed. This will help ensure that the mixture will bind together and form the sausages.
2. In a large bowl, combine the rice, beans, egg white, thyme, oregano, and sage. Stir in the onion mixture. Transfer to a food processor or blender and blend until the mixture is a solid mass, six to ten pulses. Do not puree.
3. Divide the mixture into eight parts. Roll each into a sausage shape, then roll each sausage in the panko. (If the mixture is not holding together, add a little panko until the mixture binds together into a sausage, then roll in panko.)
4. Coat a baking sheet with some of the remaining olive oil. Place the sausages on the prepared baking sheet and brush with the remaining oil. Broil until browned on all sides, for 5 to 6 minutes.

Lack of Appetite	+
Nausea, Vomiting, or Heartburn	+
Constipation	+
Diarrhea	+
Fatigue	+
Mouth Sores	+
Dry Mouth	+
Chewing or Swallowing Difficulty	+
Taste Aversion— Sweet	+
Taste Aversion— Sour & Bitter	+
Lack of Taste	+
Smells Bother	+

Nutritional Analysis: Calories 357, Total Fat 16 g, Saturated Fat 4 g, Cholesterol 156 mg, Sodium 156 mg, Carbohydrates 43 g, Dietary Fiber 6 g, Protein 11 g

Black Bean Burgers with Sun-Dried Tomatoes and Cilantro

Time: Prep: 15 minutes; Cook: 30 minutes
Serves 4 (makes 4 large or 6 to 8 small burgers)

Black beans make for a hearty vegetarian burger that eats like a regular burger. Serve on crusty bread or a hamburger bun with spicy mustard, pickles, and greens (arugula works nicely). Serve leftover burgers sans bun; add slices of avocado and top with our Tomato Habanero Salsa (page 212) or Pineapple Mango Salsa (page 213). Two very different flavors, but equally delicious with black beans!

Olive oil or nonstick cooking spray, for pan	2 tablespoons chopped fresh cilantro
2 (15-ounce) cans black beans, drained and rinsed	¾ teaspoon salt
	¼ teaspoon freshly ground black pepper
¾ cup panko or bread crumbs, plus more if needed	3 garlic cloves, minced
	Pinch of red pepper flakes
¼ cup sun-dried tomatoes, chopped	2 large eggs
	Olive oil, if needed to moisten (optional)

1. Preheat the oven to 375°F. Line a baking sheet with parchment and a bit of oil or cooking spray.
2. In a large bowl or food processor, pulse the beans until mostly mashed, while still maintaining some bits of bean.
3. Add the remaining ingredients, except the eggs and olive oil, and taste for seasoning; adjust as necessary. Add the eggs, pulse to combine, and let sit for around 15 minutes. During this time the panko will soak up a bit of the moisture. The mixture will be wet but still able to form a patty, similar to ground meat. If the mixture feels dry at all, add a bit of olive oil to moisten. If too wet, add a bit more panko.
4. Form four patties and place on the prepared baking sheet. Bake for 10 to 15 minutes on each side.

Nutritional Analysis: Calories 271, Total Fat 3 g, Saturated Fat 1 g, Cholesterol 108 mg, Sodium 427 mg, Carbohydrates 45 g, Dietary Fiber 12 g, Protein 17 g

Symptom	
Lack of Appetite	+
Nausea, Vomiting, or Heartburn	+
Constipation	+
Diarrhea	
Fatigue	+
Mouth Sores	
Dry Mouth	+
Chewing or Swallowing Difficulty	+
Taste Aversion—Sweet	+
Taste Aversion—Sour & Bitter	+
Lack of Taste	+
Smells Bother	+

Grilled Beet and Goat Cheese Burgers

Time: Prep: 15 minutes; Cook: 30 minutes
Serves 6

Lack of
Appetite

Nausea,
Vomiting, or
Heartburn

Constipation

Diarrhea

Fatigue

Mouth
Sores

Dry
Mouth

Chewing or
Swallowing
Difficulty

Taste
Aversion—
Sweet

Taste
Aversion—
Sour & Bitter

Lack of
Taste

Smells
Bother

Part of enjoying a burger is seeing that nice meaty color. Beets allow you to visually feel as if you are eating meat, when other vegetarian ingredients fall flat. Rich in folate and low in fat, beets are a great option for a vegetarian burger. Freeze raw or cooked patties in resealable plastic bags for up to a month.

4 to 5 red beets (to equal 3 cups grated beet)
1 small onion
2 garlic cloves
2 tablespoons olive oil, plus more for sautéing
2 large eggs
1½ cups rolled or quick oats, plus more

if needed
7 ounces pasteurized goat cheese or soft tofu (not silken tofu)
Handful of fresh basil, cut into thin ribbons
Pinch of salt
Pinch of freshly ground black pepper
Olive oil, for sautéing

1. Peel and grate the beets, onion, and garlic, or use a food processor to grate.
2. Place the grated vegetables in a large bowl. Add the olive oil, eggs, and oats and mix everything well.
3. Add the goat cheese, basil, salt, and pepper and stir to combine. Set aside for about 30 minutes, so the oats can soak up the liquid and the mixture sets (this step is important for the patties to hold together).
4. Shape six to eight burger patties with your hands. (If the mixture is too loose and does not hold the patty shape, add more oats.)
5. Heat 1 to 2 tablespoons of olive oil in a large skillet over medium-high heat. Add the burgers (you may need to cook in batches, depending on the size of your pan) and sauté for about 5 minutes per side, until both sides have browned.
6. Serve the burgers atop a salad or inside a bun or pita with your favorite burger toppings.

Nutritional Analysis: Calories 326, Total Fat 15 g, Saturated Fat 6 g, Cholesterol 87 mg, Sodium 333 mg, Carbohydrates 23 g, Dietary Fiber 4 g, Protein 12 g

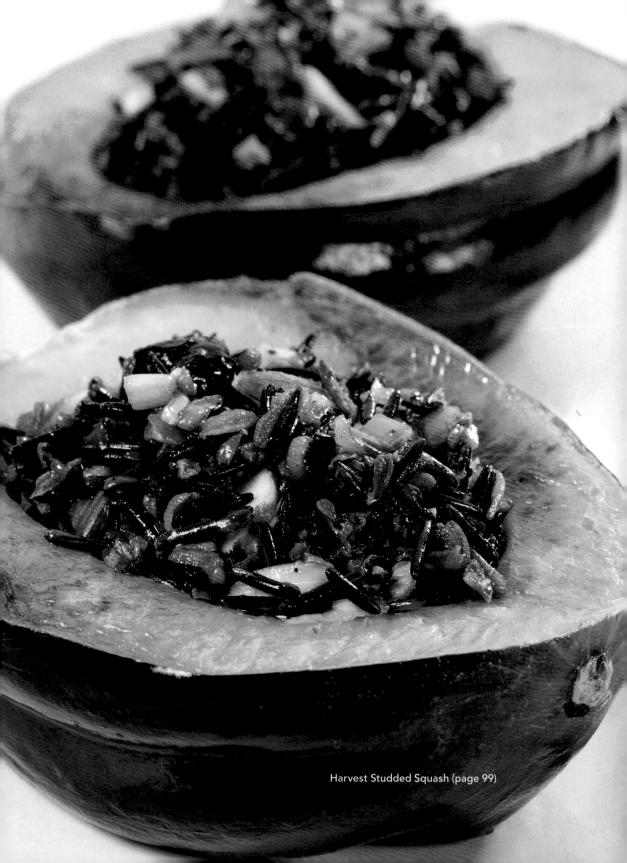

Harvest Studded Squash (page 99)

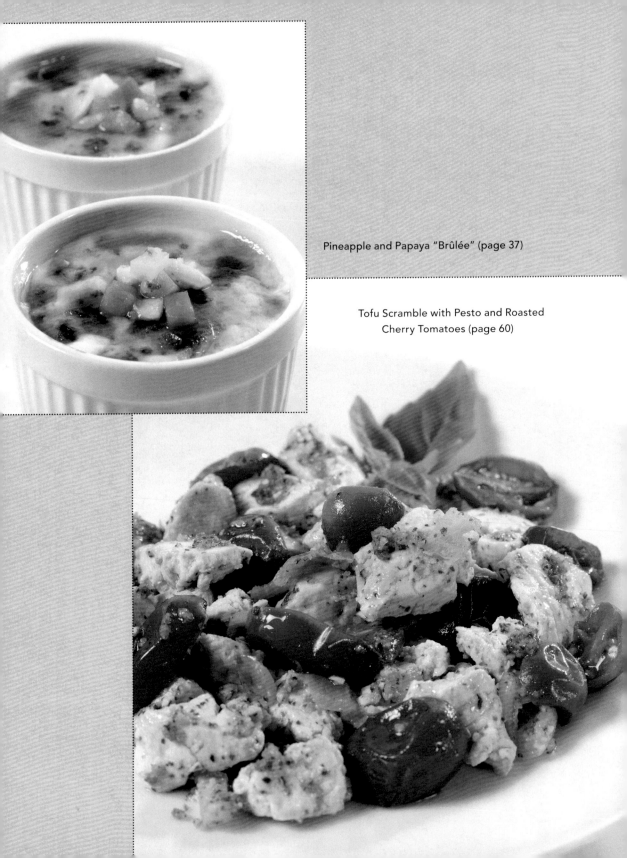

Pineapple and Papaya "Brûlée" (page 37)

Tofu Scramble with Pesto and Roasted
Cherry Tomatoes (page 60)

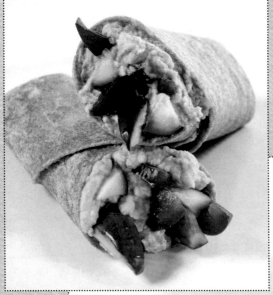

Vegetable Wraps with Edamame Spread
(page 84)

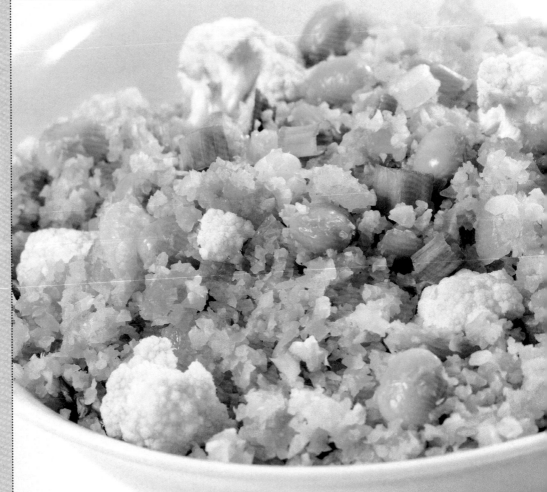

Cauliflower and Edamame "Rice" (page 182)

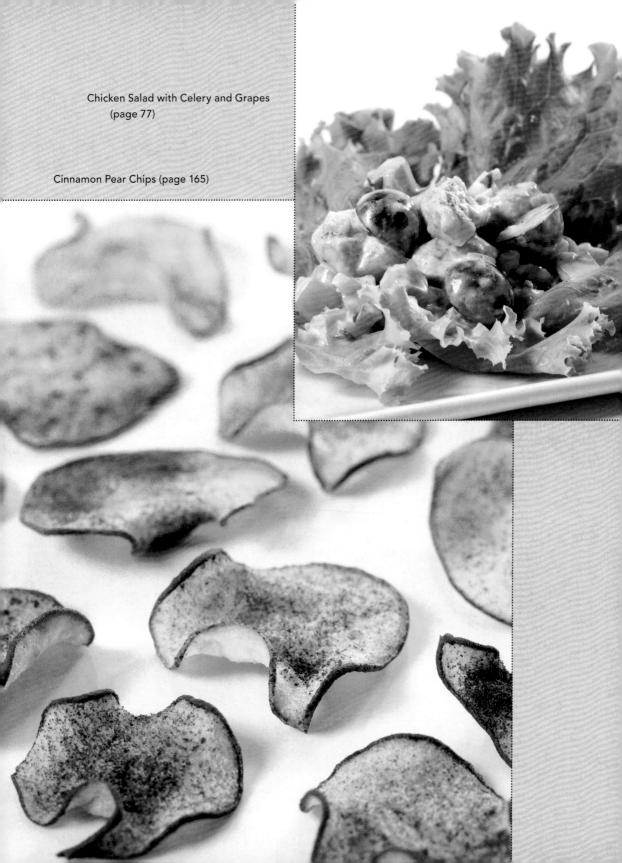

Chicken Salad with Celery and Grapes
(page 77)

Cinnamon Pear Chips (page 165)

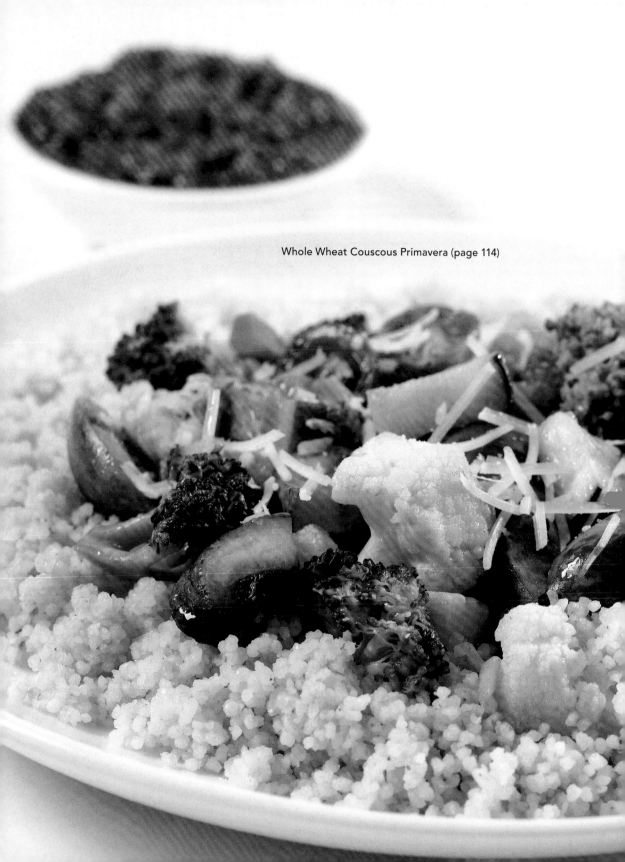

Whole Wheat Couscous Primavera (page 114)

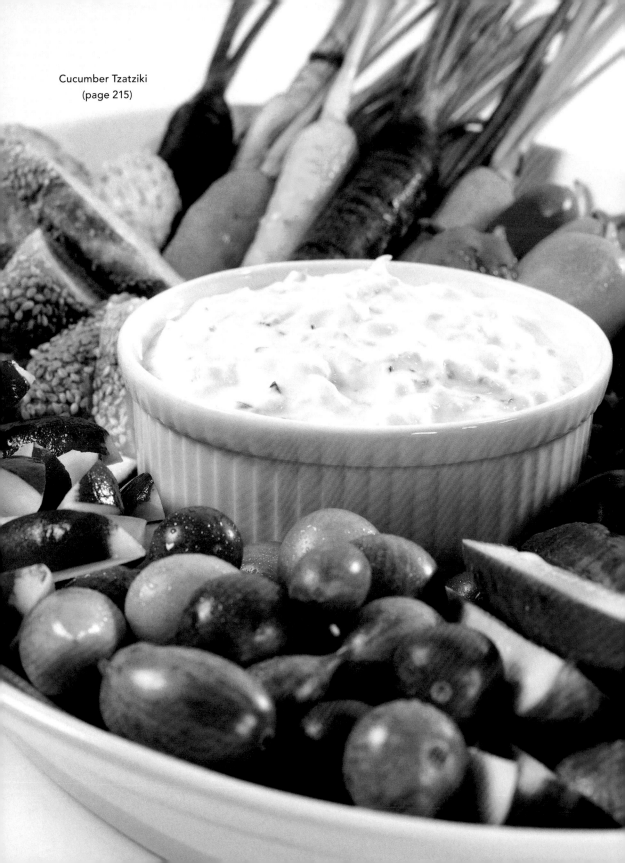

Cucumber Tzatziki
(page 215)

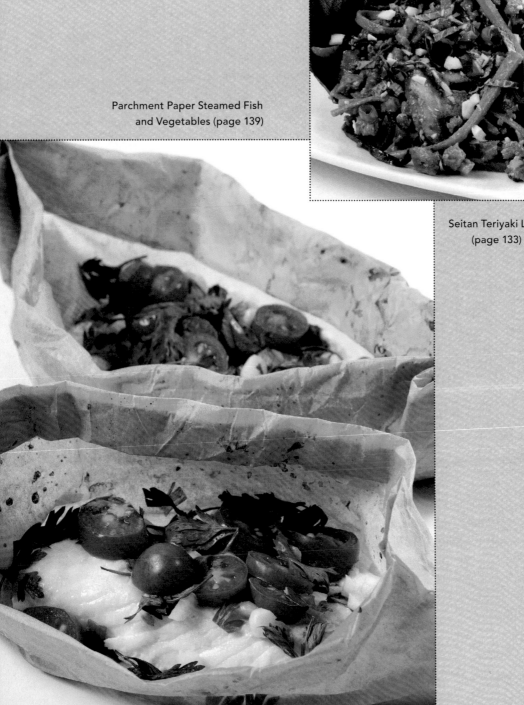

Parchment Paper Steamed Fish and Vegetables (page 139)

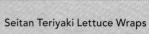

Seitan Teriyaki Lettuce Wraps (page 133)

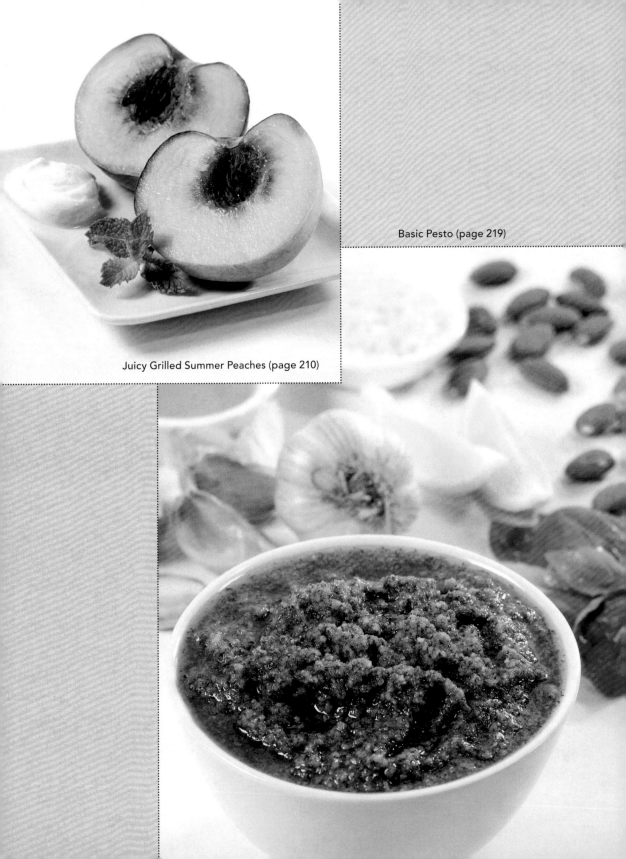

Juicy Grilled Summer Peaches (page 210)

Basic Pesto (page 219)

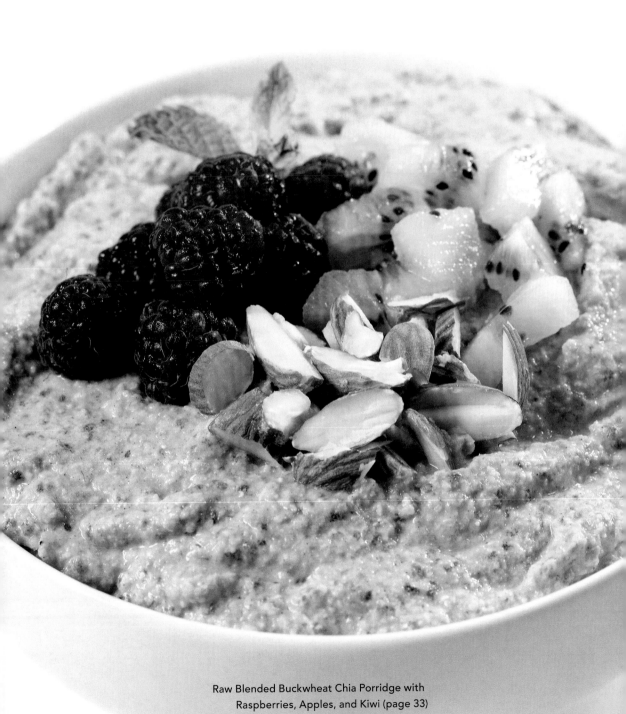

Raw Blended Buckwheat Chia Porridge with
Raspberries, Apples, and Kiwi (page 33)

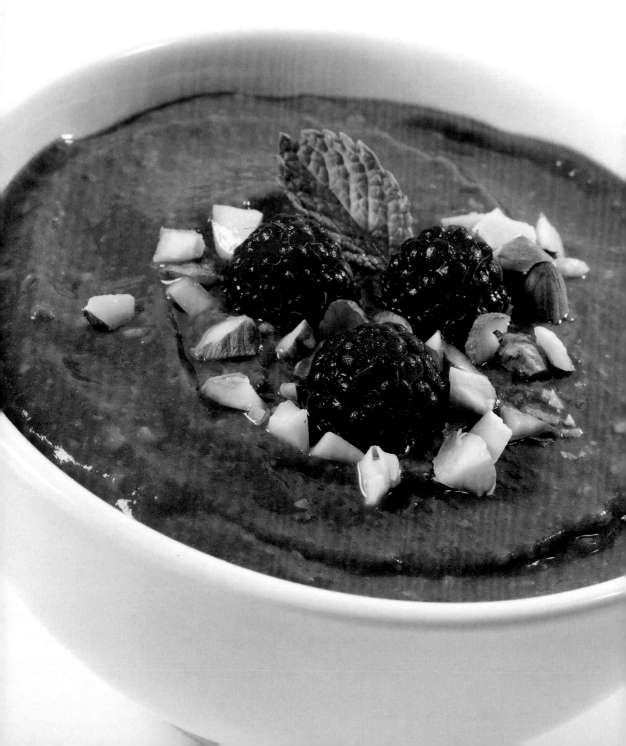

Chocolate Raspberry Pudding (page 205)

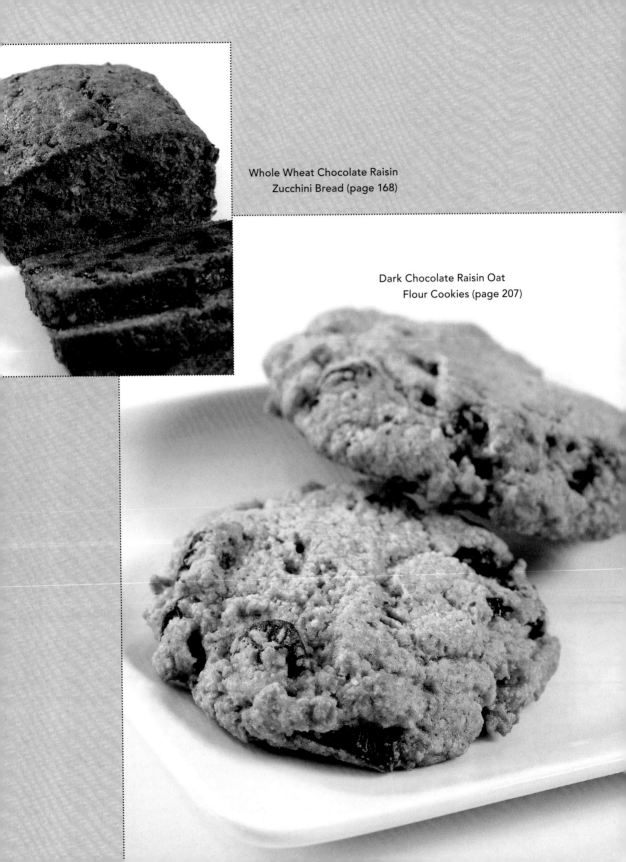

Whole Wheat Chocolate Raisin
Zucchini Bread (page 168)

Dark Chocolate Raisin Oat
Flour Cookies (page 207)

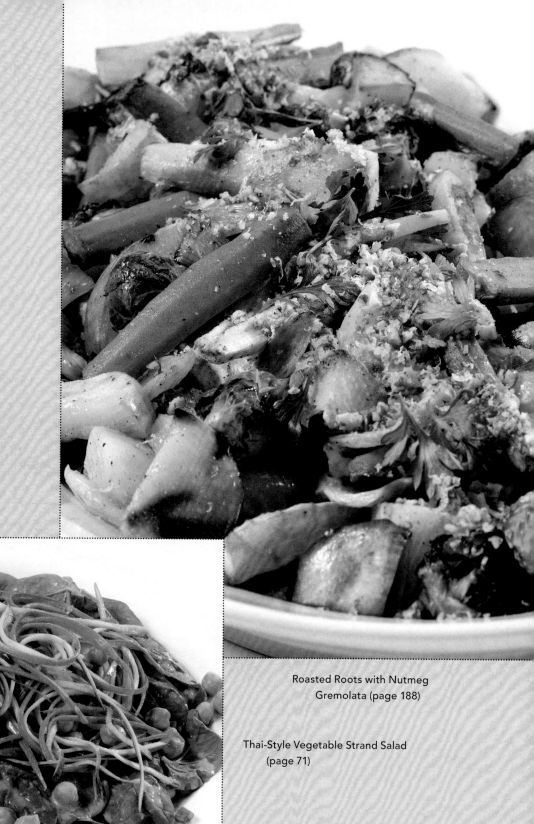

Roasted Roots with Nutmeg
Gremolata (page 188)

Thai-Style Vegetable Strand Salad
(page 71)

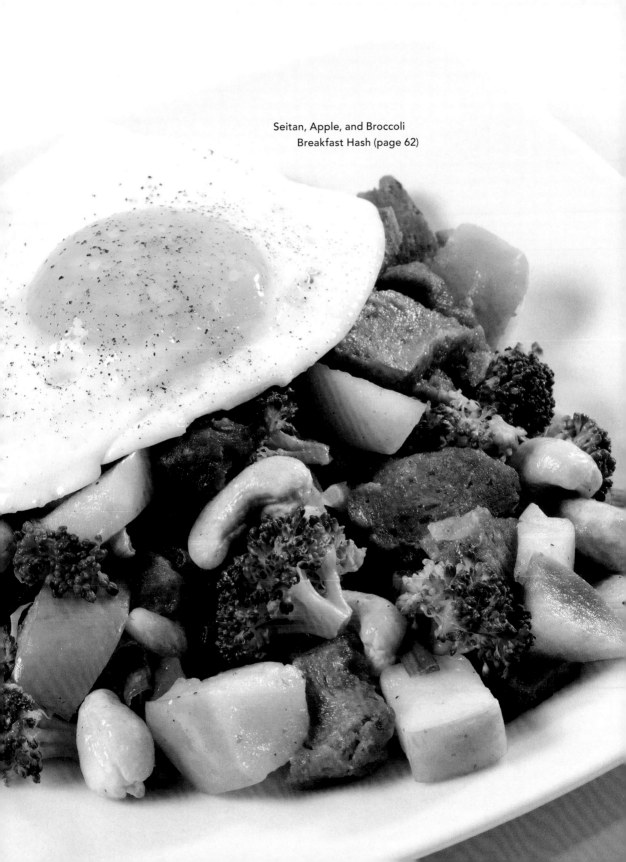

Seitan, Apple, and Broccoli
Breakfast Hash (page 62)

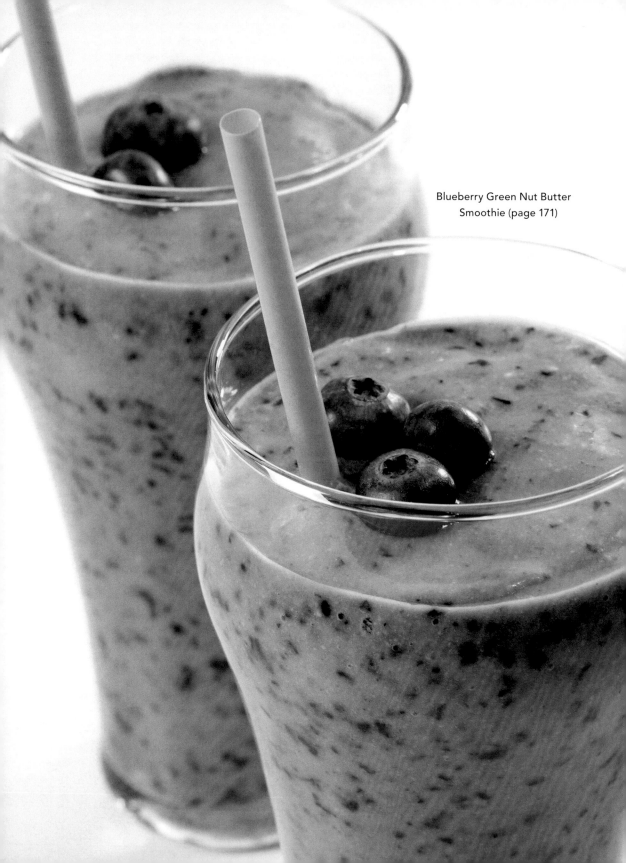

Blueberry Green Nut Butter
Smoothie (page 171)

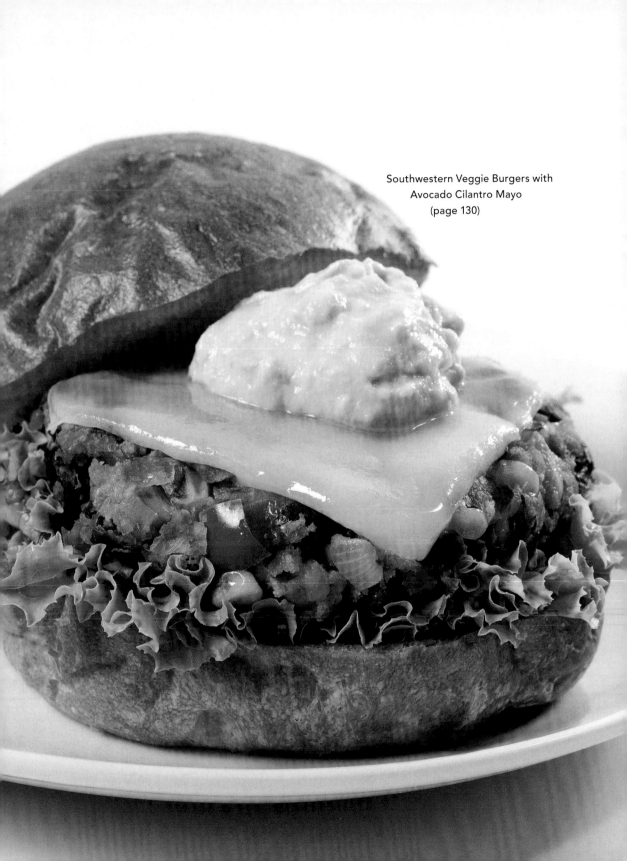

Southwestern Veggie Burgers with
Avocado Cilantro Mayo
(page 130)

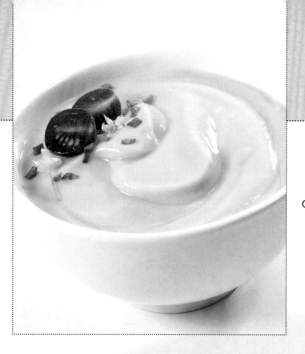

Cool Cucumber Avocado Soup
(page 149)

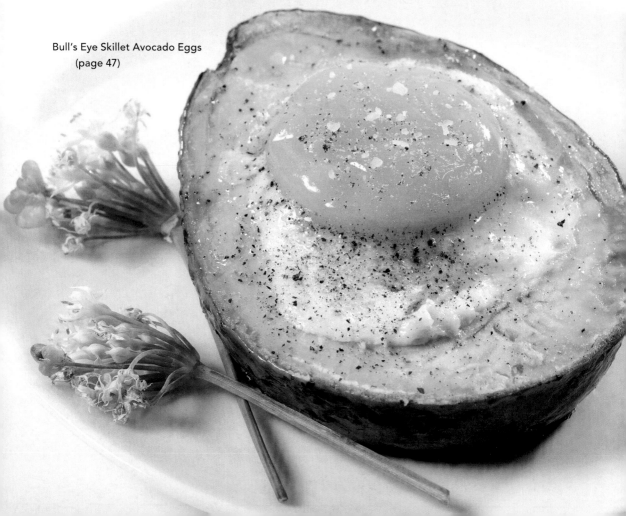

Bull's Eye Skillet Avocado Eggs
(page 47)

Balsamic Portobello Cap Burgers

Time: Prep: 15 minutes; Cook: 30 minutes
Serves 4

There is a reason portobello mushrooms make a great veggie burger; their large size and "meaty" flesh make them hearty and satisfying. For variation, try this bello burger over your favorite pasta or a whole grain instead of on a bun. If you struggle with nausea, try omitting the vinegar, onion, and tomato topping for a more neutral but still satisfying burger. If experiencing difficulty chewing or swallowing, pulse cooked mushrooms in a blender prior to eating.

2 tablespoons balsamic vinegar	4 thick slices red onion
1 tablespoon low-sodium soy sauce	4 buns
1 tablespoon olive oil, plus more for grilling	4 ounces Havarti cheese, thinly sliced
1 tablespoon chopped fresh rosemary	2 cups baby spinach
Salt and freshly ground black pepper	4 thin slices tomato
4 portobello mushroom caps, cleaned and gills removed	½ avocado, peeled, pitted, and thinly sliced

1. In a large bowl, whisk together the vinegar, soy sauce, olive oil, rosemary, and salt and pepper to taste. Place the mushroom caps in the bowl and toss with the sauce, using a spoon to evenly coat. Let stand at room temperature for 20 to 30 minutes, turning a few times.
2. Heat a grill or indoor grill pan over medium heat. When hot, brush the grate or grill pan with oil. Place the mushrooms on the grill, reserving the marinade for basting.
3. Grill for 5 to 7 minutes on each side, or until tender, brushing with marinade frequently. While the mushrooms cook, grill the onion for about 1 minute on each side and grill the buns until toasted.
4. Top the mushrooms with the cheese during the last minute of cooking.
5. To finish, place the baby spinach and grilled mushrooms on the buns and top with the grilled onion, sliced tomato, and avocado.

Nutritional Analysis: Calories 349, Total Fat 19 g, Saturated Fat 9 g, Cholesterol 35 mg, Sodium 589 mg, Carbohydrates 34 g, Dietary Fiber 5 g, Protein 14 g

Symptom	
Lack of Appetite	+
Nausea, Vomiting, or Heartburn	
Constipation	+
Diarrhea	+
Fatigue	+
Mouth Sores	
Dry Mouth	+
Chewing or Swallowing Difficulty	+
Taste Aversion—Sweet	+
Taste Aversion—Sour & Bitter	
Lack of Taste	+
Smells Bother	+

Southwestern Veggie Burgers with Avocado Cilantro Mayo ⓘ

Time: Prep: 15 minutes; Cook: 15 minutes
Serves 6

+	Lack of Appetite
	Nausea, Vomiting, or Heartburn
+	Constipation
	Diarrhea
+	Fatigue
	Mouth Sores
+	Dry Mouth
+	Chewing or Swallowing Difficulty
+	Taste Aversion— Sweet
+	Taste Aversion— Sour & Bitter
+	Lack of Taste
+	Smells Bother

This is a bright and colorful alternative to the more brown-colored, grain-based veggie burgers, but equally satisfying. In addition to, or instead of, the avocado mayo, try topping them with salsa and Jack cheese; or enjoy just as they are hot off the pan. If sensitive to spice, omit the hot sauce and reduce the garlic in the avocado mayo. Leftover avocado cilantro mayo tastes great when spread over warm corn bread, added to homemade burritos and tacos, or drizzled over roasted potatoes.

1 (15-ounce) can black beans, drained and rinsed
4 tablespoons olive oil
1 medium-size onion, diced
½ medium-size red bell pepper, seeded and diced
½ cup fresh, frozen, or canned corn (thawed if using frozen, drained if using canned)
1 medium-size jicama, diced
Salt and freshly ground black pepper
1 cup panko or bread crumbs
½ cup salsa

6 slices Jack cheese
6 buns

For the avocado cilantro mayo
1 avocado, peeled and pitted
2 tablespoons finely chopped fresh cilantro
½ cup plain Greek yogurt
1 to 2 garlic cloves, minced
½ tablespoon hot sauce, or more to taste
½ tablespoon freshly squeezed lime juice
Salt

1. In a large bowl or food processor, mash three quarters of the beans. This should not be a puree, but more of a mush so you should still see some parts of the beans. Once done, add the remaining beans to this mush and mix together.

2. In a large skillet, heat 2 tablespoons of the oil over medium heat. Add the onion and sauté for 5 minutes, or until it starts to soften.

3. Add the bell pepper, corn, and jicama and sauté for 3 to 5 minutes, until the jicama begins to soften. Season with salt and black pepper to taste.

4. Remove from the heat and add to the beans. Add the panko and fold in the salsa until everything is combined.
5. Divide the mixture into six equal parts and form patties.
6. Wipe the skillet clean. Heat the remaining 2 tablespoons of oil in the skillet over medium heat and cook the patties on one side until golden, for 2 to 3 minutes. Flip carefully and cook until golden, for another 2 to 3 minutes. Top the burgers with the cheese in the last minute of cooking.
7. Make the avocado cilantro mayo: Mash together the avocado, cilantro, yogurt, garlic, hot sauce, lime juice, and salt. Taste and adjust the seasonings to your liking.
8. To serve, place the patties in the buns and top with the avocado cilantro mayo.

Nutritional Analysis (burgers): Calories 424, Total Fat 18 g, Saturated Fat 6 g, Cholesterol 20 mg, Sodium 439 mg, Carbohydrates 49 g, Dietary Fiber 6 g, Protein 15 g

Nutritional Analysis (avocado cilantro mayo): Calories 67, Total Fat 5 g, Saturated Fat 1 g, Cholesterol 1 mg, Sodium 49 mg, Carbohydrates 4 g, Dietary Fiber 2 g, Protein 2 g

Chickpea Flour Pizza Margherita

Time: Prep: 15 minutes; Cook: 30 minutes
Serves 2

Lack of
Appetite

Nausea,
Vomiting, or
Heartburn

Constipation

Diarrhea

Fatigue

Mouth
Sores

Dry
Mouth

Chewing or
Swallowing
Difficulty

Taste
Aversion—
Sweet

Taste
Aversion—
Sour & Bitter

Lack of
Taste

Smells
Bother

Chickpea flour is soft and fine like all-purpose flour but has a subtle nutty flavor and a little extra protein. Add your favorite toppings to make different pizzas or twist the dough into breadsticks and dip in our Mirepoix Marinara Sauce (page 217). Serve with light or no tomato sauce for nausea or mouth soreness. The dough will last in the refrigerator for 3 to 4 days.

1 tablespoon olive oil, plus more for pan

½ cup warm water (about 110°F)

1 teaspoon fast-acting yeast

½ teaspoon honey

1¼ cups chickpea flour

¼ teaspoon garlic powder

¼ teaspoon onion powder

½ cup tomato sauce

1 cup shredded mozzarella cheese

Fresh basil leaves, for topping

1. Preheat the oven to 475°F. Coat a 12-inch pizza pan with olive oil.
2. In large bowl, combine the warm water, yeast, oil, and honey. Stir to dissolve the yeast. Add the chickpea flour, garlic powder, and onion powder. Mix thoroughly. Let the dough rest for 5 minutes.
3. Place the dough on the prepared pizza pan and spread until it covers the pan, leaving a 1-inch border. Add the tomato sauce, leaving ½-inch border uncovered. Sprinkle with the cheese.
4. Bake for 12 minutes. Remove from the oven, dot with basil leaves, and let cool for a few minutes.

Nutritional Analysis: Calories 524, Total Fat 23 g, Saturated Fat 8 g, Cholesterol 30 mg, Sodium 676 mg, Carbohydrates 53 g, Dietary Fiber 16 g, Protein 33 g

Seitan Teriyaki Lettuce Wraps ①

Time: 30 minutes
Serves 4

The seitan and sauce give these vegetarian lettuce wraps an irresistible umami flavor, while the colorful veggies lend a refreshing crunch in every bite. Lettuce wraps are an easy and inexpensive way to cut down on carbs and calories, if needed. Chopped chicken or turkey breast can be used as alternative proteins. If experiencing difficulty chewing or swallowing, pulse cooked seitan sauté in a blender prior to eating.

1 teaspoon olive oil
4 garlic cloves, minced
1 (1-inch) piece fresh ginger, grated
4 ounces seitan, finely chopped
1 medium-size carrot, cut into small
   matchsticks
6 small mushrooms, thinly sliced
¼ small head red cabbage, shredded
2 scallions, sliced

2 tablespoons freshly squeezed
   lime juice
2 tablespoons low-sodium soy sauce
Pinch of chili powder
2 tablespoons teriyaki sauce
1 large egg
½ head iceberg or butter lettuce
Dry-roasted peanuts, crushed

1. In a large skillet, heat the olive oil over medium heat. Add the garlic and ginger and sauté for a minute.
2. Add the seitan, carrot, mushrooms, cabbage, and scallions and sauté for another minute (if the pan gets dry, add a little water). Mix in the lime juice, soy sauce, chili powder, and teriyaki sauce.
3. Push the ingredients to the side and crack the egg in the skillet. Stir quickly to break the yolk and then incorporate the egg with the rest of the mixture. Once the egg is cooked, remove the skillet from the heat.
4. Assemble by filling a whole piece of lettuce with 2 to 3 tablespoons of the seitan mixture and then sprinkle crushed peanuts on top.

Nutritional Analysis (not including crushed peanuts): Calories 124, Total Fat 3 g, Saturated Fat 1 g, Cholesterol 54 mg, Sodium 744 mg, Carbohydrates 14 g, Dietary Fiber 2 g, Protein 12 g

Lack of Appetite +
Nausea, Vomiting, or Heartburn
Constipation +
Diarrhea
Fatigue +
Mouth Sores
Dry Mouth +
Chewing or Swallowing Difficulty +
Taste Aversion— Sweet
Taste Aversion— Sour & Bitter
Lack of Taste +
Smells Bother +

Tempeh Kebabs with Homemade Barbecue Sauce

Time: Prep: 15 minutes; Cook: 30 minutes
Serves 8

Lack of
Appetite

Nausea,
Vomiting, or
Heartburn

Constipation

Diarrhea

Fatigue

Mouth
Sores

Dry
Mouth

Chewing or
Swallowing
Difficulty

Taste
Aversion—
Sweet

Taste
Aversion—
Sour & Bitter

Lack of
Taste

Smells
Bother

These kebabs offer a double dose of phytonutrients from the soy-based tempeh and fresh vegetables. Try the barbecue sauce warm and see how the flavors change. For a time saver, use your favorite bottle of barbecue sauce. Serve leftovers on a bed of Red Cabbage Slaw (page 75) or stuffed into a bun for a barbecued tempeh sandwich.

For the barbecue sauce

1 (15-ounce) can tomato sauce
2 tablespoons pure maple
    syrup
1 tablespoon molasses
2 tablespoons olive oil
2 tablespoons low-sodium
    soy sauce
1 tablespoon cider vinegar
2 tablespoons grated ginger
1 cup chopped cilantro
1 teaspoon chili powder
Pinch of red pepper flakes

For the tempeh

2 (8-ounce) packages tempeh,
    cut into 1½-inch pieces
2 medium-size yellow or orange bell
    peppers, seeded and cut into
    1½-inch pieces
1 medium-size zucchini, cut into
    1½-inch pieces
1 medium-size white or yellow onion,
    cut into 1½-inch pieces
8 ounces white mushrooms,
    washed and trimmed

1. Whisk together all the barbecue sauce ingredients. Pour the sauce into a 9 by 9-inch or 9 by 13-inch casserole dish.
2. Add the tempeh and vegetables, coat well with the sauce, and allow them to marinate in the refrigerator for at least 2 hours or overnight.
3. Soak wooden or bamboo skewers in water for at least 20 minutes (this is to prevent their burning on the grill). Divide the vegetables and tempeh evenly onto the soaked skewers, alternating ingredients. Reserve some extra sauce for serving.
4. Heat a grill to medium-high heat. Place the skewers on the grill and cook, basting occasionally, for 7 to 10 minutes, or until the vegetables are tender and everything is browned. Alternatively, you can use a grill pan, cooking for 8 to 10 minutes on medium-high heat. Serve immediately.

Nutritional Analysis (kebabs): Calories 142, Total Fat 4 g, Saturated Fat 1 g, Cholesterol 0 mg, Sodium 10 mg, Carbohydrates 13 g, Dietary Fiber 7 g, Protein 12 g

Nutritional Analysis (per ¼ cup barbecue sauce): Calories 59, Total Fat 3 g, Saturated Fat 0 g, Cholesterol 0 mg, Sodium 341 mg, Carbohydrates 8 g, Dietary Fiber 1 g, Protein 1 g

Baked Tofu and Broccoli over Wild Rice

Time: Prep: 15 minutes; Cook: 30 minutes
Serves 4

+	Lack of Appetite
	Nausea, Vomiting, or Heartburn
+	Constipation
	Diarrhea
+	Fatigue
+	Mouth Sores
+	Dry Mouth
	Chewing or Swallowing Difficulty
+	Taste Aversion— Sweet
+	Taste Aversion— Sour & Bitter
+	Lack of Taste
+	Smells Bother

Wild rice has a different texture and taste than white or brown rice because it is actually a grass. As such, using wild rice is a fun way to change up a meal if you are tired of regular or brown rice. If you are experiencing diarrhea or nausea, try replacing the broccoli with well-cooked zucchini or squash and substitute mild white basmati rice. Sauté leftovers in a pan with a beaten egg to make a quick fried rice.

For the tofu and broccoli

2 tablespoons balsamic vinegar

1 tablespoon olive oil

1 tablespoon agave nectar or honey

1 garlic clove, minced

¼ teaspoon dried oregano

¼ teaspoon dried thyme

Salt and freshly ground black pepper

1 (14-ounce) package extra-firm tofu

5 cups medium-dice broccoli or frozen broccoli florets

For the wild rice

1 cup uncooked wild rice, rinsed

½ tablespoon olive oil

¼ teaspoon salt

1. Begin the tofu and broccoli: Combine the balsamic vinegar, olive oil, agave nectar, garlic, oregano, thyme, salt, and pepper in a bowl.
2. Drain the tofu and gently press to remove as much liquid as possible. Cut the tofu into cubes. Pierce the tofu in several places with a fork to allow the flavor to permeate the tofu.
3. Pour the balsamic mixture over the tofu and marinate for 30 minutes to an hour.
4. While the tofu marinates, make the wild rice: Combine the wild rice, oil, salt, and 2 cups of water in a medium-size saucepan. Place the pan over high heat and bring to a boil.
5. Lower the heat to a simmer and cook, covered, until the wild rice is tender and there is no water left in the pot, for about 1 hour. If the rice is cooked and there is still liquid left in the pan, drain the water out of the rice.
6. Preheat the oven to 400°F. Spread the marinated tofu on a shallow 9 by 13-inch baking pan. Save any leftover marinade for the broccoli.

7. Cover with foil and bake for 20 minutes. Uncover the tofu, add the broccoli, and bake for 10 minutes more. Turn the tofu and continue to bake for an additional 10 minutes.
8. If the tofu is not browned enough for you, turn on your broiler and broil the tofu for 5 minutes, monitoring closely. Then turn the tofu pieces and broil for another 5 minutes.
9. Mix with the wild rice or serve on the side and enjoy.

Nutritional Analysis: Calories 334, Total Fat 11 g, Saturated Fat 2 g, Cholesterol 0 mg, Sodium 153 mg, Carbohydrates 43 g, Dietary Fiber 7 g, Protein 19 g

Panfried Tofu and Vegetables over Brown Rice

Time: Prep: 15 minutes; Cook: 30 minutes
Serves 6

This warm dish is a little sweet, a little tart, and a little savory all in one and is perfect for lunch or dinner. And no need to limit the grain to just rice; try it over any whole grain, such as farro or barley, and see what you like best. Chicken, turkey, or shrimp can be easily substituted for tofu.

1½ cups uncooked brown rice	1 cup chopped asparagus
¼ cup teriyaki sauce	1 cup chopped mushrooms
¼ cup low-sodium soy sauce	1 cup chopped zucchini
1 (14-ounce) package extra-firm tofu	1 cup shredded carrot
2 tablespoons canola oil	3 scallions, minced

1. Cook the rice according to the package directions.
2. Combine the teriyaki and soy sauce in a small dish or measuring cup to make a stir-fry sauce.
3. Cut the tofu into slices and press with a paper towel to remove excess moisture. Wait a few minutes and press again. Cut the tofu slices into small cubes.
4. Heat the canola oil in a large, nonstick skillet over medium heat.
5. Add the tofu and about ¼ cup of the stir-fry sauce. Panfry the tofu until golden brown. Remove from the pan and drain on paper towel–lined plates.
6. Return the pan to the heat and place the asparagus, mushrooms, and zucchini in the pan with the remaining stir-fry sauce. When the asparagus is bright green and tender-crisp, add the carrot and toss together.
7. Arrange the veggies and tofu over the cooked rice, and sprinkle with the scallions.

Nutritional Analysis: Calories 315, Total Fat 10 g, Saturated Fat 1 g, Cholesterol 0 mg, Sodium 786 mg, Carbohydrates 44 g, Dietary Fiber 4 g, Protein 13 g

Lack of Appetite

Nausea, Vomiting, or Heartburn

Constipation

Diarrhea

Fatigue

Mouth Sores

Dry Mouth

Chewing or Swallowing Difficulty

Taste Aversion— Sweet

Taste Aversion— Sour & Bitter

Lack of Taste

Smells Bother

Parchment Paper Steamed Fish and Vegetables

Time: Prep: 15 minutes; Cook: 30 minutes
Serves 4

Steaming fish makes it moist and tender and therefore one of the most perfect soft meals for those with difficulty chewing and swallowing and mouth sores. This recipe is truly easy and quick for those in need of a time-saving meal and there is very little cleanup! Substitute zucchini or squash for the tomatoes if experiencing mouth sores. This fish pairs well with Sautéed Asparagus and Peas (page 186) or Glazed Brussels Sprouts (page 181).

1½ pounds mild white fish, such as cod, tilapia, or halibut	6 cherry or grape tomatoes, halved
Zest of 1 lemon	Juice of 1 lemon
1 scallion, chopped	¼ teaspoon salt
2 garlic cloves, minced	¼ teaspoon freshly ground black pepper
	¼ cup chopped fresh parsley

1. Preheat the oven to 375°F. Line a baking sheet with parchment paper. Fold the parchment paper in half, then open it back up and place the fish on one half, close to the crease.
2. Combine the remaining ingredients and place on top of and around the fish.
3. Fold the other half of the parchment over the top of the fish and vegetables. Working around the edges, fold the parchment over tightly in ¼-inch folds, then fold up the ends to make a closed packet. Bake for 12 to 15 minutes. Remove from the oven.
4. Place on a plate and carefully remove the fish from the paper and serve.

Nutritional Analysis: Calories 152, Total Fat 1 g, Saturated Fat 0 g, Cholesterol 73 mg, Sodium 216 mg, Carbohydrates 3 g, Dietary Fiber 1 g, Protein 31 g

Lack of Appetite	+
Nausea, Vomiting, or Heartburn	+
Constipation	+
Diarrhea	+
Fatigue	+
Mouth Sores	
Dry Mouth	+
Chewing or Swallowing Difficulty	+
Taste Aversion—Sweet	+
Taste Aversion—Sour & Bitter	+
Lack of Taste	+
Smells Bother	+

Greek Grilled Salmon with Tzatziki Sauce

Time: Prep: 15 minutes; Cook: 30 minutes
Serves 4

Choose wild salmon rather than farmed salmon as the best source of heart-healthy omega-3 fatty acids (wild caught salmon has a bright pink/fuchsia color to the flesh, whereas farmed salmon will be lighter pink or orangey). Make Greek pita sandwiches with leftovers: Take a pita and fill it with salmon, tzatziki sauce, and chopped vegetables, such as cucumber and tomato. Toss in some Supersmooth Ginger Hummus (page 223) for an extra boost of Mediterranean flavor.

Juice and zest of 1 lemon

3 garlic cloves, roughly chopped

1 teaspoon dried oregano

½ teaspoon salt

½ teaspoon freshly ground black pepper

1½ pounds skinless salmon fillet, ½ inch thick

1 tablespoon olive oil, for grill or skillet

½ cup Cucumber Tzatziki (page 215)

1. Mix together the lemon juice and zest, garlic, oregano, salt, and pepper. Place the salmon in a large bowl or container with a lid. Pour the marinade over the salmon and cover the bowl or container.
2. Let the salmon marinate for at least 15 minutes or for several hours in the fridge.
3. Once marinated, heat the oil on the grill or skillet over medium-high heat. Add the salmon and cook for about 4 minutes per side, or until the fish is just cooked through and opaque inside.
4. Serve with a large scoop of tzatziki sauce.

Nutritional Analysis (with 2 tablespoons Cucumber Tzatziki per serving):
Calories 387, Total Fat 25 g, Saturated Fat 6 g, Cholesterol 96 mg, Sodium 508 mg, Carbohydrates 3 g, Dietary Fiber 0 g, Protein 37 g

Lack of Appetite

Nausea, Vomiting, or Heartburn

Constipation

Diarrhea

Fatigue

Mouth Sores

Dry Mouth

Chewing or Swallowing Difficulty

Taste Aversion— Sweet

Taste Aversion— Sour & Bitter

Lack of Taste

Smells Bother

Maitake Mushroom and Tomato Poached Salmon

Time: Prep: 15 minutes; Cook: 30 minutes
Serves 2

Try this dish over brown rice or soba noodles and shake a few toasted sesame seeds on top for extra-special presentation (an extra teaspoon of sesame oil never hurt, either). To combat nausea, reduce or omit some of the ingredients as needed, but keep the ginger, which has excellent stomach-soothing and anti-nausea properties. To make it vegetarian, swap out the fish fillet for a block of tofu, sliced in half lengthwise.

1 teaspoon sesame oil	1 cup sliced maitake mushrooms
2 garlic cloves, smashed	1 large tomato, sliced
1 (1-inch) piece fresh ginger, peeled and minced	2 cups chopped bok choy
	2 (6-ounce) salmon fillets
½ medium-size red onion, thinly sliced	Salt and freshly ground black pepper

1. Heat a medium-size pan over high heat.
2. When the pan is hot, slowly stir in the sesame oil and garlic and ginger. When an aroma releases, lower the heat and add the onion and then the maitake mushrooms. Add a little water and steam the vegetables for about 2 minutes.
3. Layer on the tomato, then the bok choy, and lastly the salmon. Season the salmon with salt and pepper.
4. Cover tightly with a lid. Keeping the heat on low, cook for 10 to 15 minutes, or until the salmon is fully cooked and can easily be flaked with a fork.

Nutritional Analysis: Calories 454, Total Fat 26 g, Saturated Fat 6 g, Cholesterol 94 mg, Sodium 162 mg, Carbohydrates 17 g, Dietary Fiber 5 g, Protein 40 g

Nutritionist's Favorite to Savor
This is my favorite because so many people ask me how to include healthful immune-boosting maitake mushrooms in their diet and this is a perfect way to complement and flavor salmon, or any fish that you enjoy cooking.

Lack of Appetite	+
Nausea, Vomiting, or Heartburn	
Constipation	+
Diarrhea	+
Fatigue	+
Mouth Sores	
Dry Mouth	+
Chewing or Swallowing Difficulty	+
Taste Aversion— Sweet	+
Taste Aversion— Sour & Bitter	+
Lack of Taste	+
Smells Bother	

Moist and Tender Whole Sea Bass on the Grill

Time: Prep: 15 minutes; Cook: 30 minutes
Serves 6

Sea bass is a mild white fish that allows the subtle Mediterranean flavors of the seasoning to shine. Like most seafood, sea bass is a great source of lean protein and healthy, unsaturated fats, which can help improve your cholesterol, decrease your risk of heart disease, and reduce inflammation.

1 (3-pound) whole sea bass, butterflied	5 sprigs rosemary
4 to 6 teaspoons olive oil	10 sprigs thyme
Salt and freshly ground black pepper	10 sprigs oregano
½ medium-size red onion, thinly sliced	6 lemon wedges, for garnish
3 garlic cloves, thinly sliced	Additional herbs, for garnish

1. Wash and pat dry the fish.
2. Open the fish. Spread the interior with 2 to 3 teaspoons of the olive oil and season with salt and pepper.
3. Evenly spread out the onion, garlic, rosemary, thyme, and oregano sprigs inside the fish. Close the fish.
4. Spread 2 to 3 teaspoons of olive oil on the skin of the fish, top and bottom, and season with salt and pepper.
5. Wrap the fish in foil, leaving an accessible opening at the top so that you can check for doneness.
6. Heat a grill to medium heat, then place the wrapped fish on the grill, closing the top of the grill. After 10 minutes, open the foil and check the fish with a fork. When the fish is a solid white throughout, remove it from the grill. Depending on the heat of the grill, and the thickness of the fish, the cooking time will vary from 10 to 15 minutes.
7. Open the foil. With a large, flat spatula, remove the fish from the foil and place on a platter.
8. Place lemon wedges and extra herbs around the fish, for garnish.

Nutritional Analysis: Calories 250, Total Fat 8 g, Saturated Fat 2 g, Cholesterol 93 mg, Sodium 235 mg, Carbohydrates 1 g, Dietary Fiber 0 g, Protein 42 g

Lack of Appetite

Nausea, Vomiting, or Heartburn

Constipation

Diarrhea

Fatigue

Mouth Sores

Dry Mouth

Chewing or Swallowing Difficulty

Taste Aversion— Sweet

Taste Aversion— Sour & Bitter

Lack of Taste

Smells Bother

Chicken Ropa Vieja

Time: Prep: 15 minutes; Cook: 1 hour
Serves 6

Ropa vieja, meaning "old clothes," is a popular dish in Cuban cuisine, traditionally prepared with red meat. Chicken is used here to lighten up the calories. Garlic and cumin are the flavor backbones, so feel free to adjust their amounts to your liking. Turn leftovers into enchiladas by filling corn tortillas with the chicken mixture, covering with extra sauce or salsa, and baking until heated through.

To poach

3 (8-ounce) skinless, boneless chicken breasts

1 small onion, diced

1 tomato, diced

1 carrot, peeled and chopped

2 garlic cloves, sliced and diced

Salt

To finish

1 tablespoon olive oil

2 garlic cloves

1 small onion, sliced

1 medium-size green bell pepper, seeded and sliced

1 medium-size red bell pepper, seeded and sliced

½ cup tomato sauce

1 teaspoon ground cumin

¼ teaspoon garlic powder

½ teaspoon salt, plus more to taste

¼ teaspoon freshly ground black pepper, plus more to taste

Cooked brown rice, for serving

1. Poach the chicken: Place the chicken, onion, tomato, carrot, garlic, and a big pinch of salt in a large pot. Add just enough water to cover. Bring to a boil, then lower the heat to a bare simmer and poach for about 30 minutes, or until the chicken is tender and cooked through. Alternatively, place everything in a slow cooker and cook on HIGH for 4 hours, or until the chicken is tender.
2. When done, remove the chicken and shred with two forks; set aside. Reserve 1 cup of the poaching liquid and save the rest to use in other recipes.
3. Finish the dish: In a large, deep skillet, heat the olive oil over medium heat. Add the garlic, onion, and bell peppers. Cook for 3 to 4 minutes, or until soft.

Symptom	
Lack of Appetite	+
Nausea, Vomiting, or Heartburn	+
Constipation	+
Diarrhea	
Fatigue	+
Mouth Sores	
Dry Mouth	+
Chewing or Swallowing Difficulty	+
Taste Aversion— Sweet	+
Taste Aversion— Sour & Bitter	+
Lack of Taste	+
Smells Bother	+

4. Stir in the cooked chicken, tomato sauce, and 1 cup of the reserved chicken poaching liquid. Add the cumin, garlic powder, salt, and black pepper.
5. Cover and simmer over low heat for 8 to 10 minutes, adding more poaching liquid and seasoning, if needed.
6. Serve over brown rice.

Nutritional Analysis (not including rice): Calories 174, Total Fat 5 g, Saturated Fat 1 g, Cholesterol 73 mg, Sodium 413 mg, Carbohydrates 5 g, Dietary Fiber 1 g, Protein 25 g

Cilantro Chicken Fajitas ①

Time: Prep: 15 minutes; Cook: 15 minutes
Serves 4

The cilantro lime marinade is the star of this fajita dish and would work equally well over shrimp or a mild white fish. For a vegetarian option, substitute strips of tofu.

2 (8-ounce) chicken breasts

¼ cup + 1 tablespoon olive oil

3 tablespoons freshly squeezed lime juice

2 tablespoons teriyaki or soy sauce

½ teaspoon ground cumin

½ teaspoon dried oregano

⅛ teaspoon cayenne pepper or red pepper flakes

2 garlic cloves, pressed or grated

2 tablespoons chopped fresh cilantro, plus more for garnish

1 medium-size red onion, cut into ¼-inch slices

1 medium-size red bell pepper, seeded and cut into ¼-inch slices

1 medium-size green bell pepper, seeded and cut into ¼-inch slices

Salt and freshly ground black pepper

8 (6-inch) corn tortillas

1. Cut the chicken into ¼ by 2-inch strips.
2. Whisk together ¼ cup of the olive oil with the lime juice, teriyaki sauce, cumin, oregano, cayenne, garlic, and cilantro.
3. Place the chicken in a plastic container, resealable plastic bag, or large bowl. Pour the marinade over the chicken and toss to coat thoroughly. Cover and refrigerate for 2 to 12 hours, stirring or gently shaking the container occasionally.
4. Heat the remaining tablespoon of olive oil in a large, cast-iron skillet over medium-high heat. Add the onion and bell peppers and cook for about 5 minutes, stirring occasionally, until the vegetables are just tender and fragrant. Transfer the vegetables to a plate and set aside.
5. Place the skillet back on medium-high heat and place half of the chicken in the pan. Cook for 5 minutes, flip, and cook for 5 minutes more. Add to the plate of cooked vegetables. Cook the remaining chicken. Toss all the cooked chicken together with the vegetables and a pinch each of salt and black pepper.
6. Heat the tortillas directly over the flame of a gas stove or in a dry non-stick pan for a few seconds.

Lack of Appetite	+
Nausea, Vomiting, or Heartburn	
Constipation	+
Diarrhea	
Fatigue	+
Mouth Sores	
Dry Mouth	+
Chewing or Swallowing Difficulty	+
Taste Aversion— Sweet	+
Taste Aversion— Sour & Bitter	+
Lack of Taste	+
Smells Bother	+

7. Place two tortillas on each plate. Top evenly with the chicken mixture, garnish with cilantro, and enjoy.

Nutritional Analysis: Calories 399, Total Fat 21 g, Saturated Fat 3 g, Cholesterol 73 mg, Sodium 451 mg, Carbohydrates 24 g, Dietary Fiber 4 g, Protein 28 g

Stretch and Save: Make nachos! Cut leftover tortillas into triangles, spread on a parchment-lined baking sheet and bake in a 350°F oven with a touch of olive oil and salt for 10 to 15 minutes, to make your own tortilla chips. Top the chips with leftover fajita filling and return them to the oven for another 10 to 15 minutes. Top with salsa and sour cream.

Turkey and Oat Meat Loaf

Time: Prep: 15 minutes; Cook: 45 minutes
Serves 8

This is comfort food at its finest. Oats help to bind the loaf and give a little extra fiber along the way. As a time-saver and for those with less energy, make the meat loaf ahead in muffin tins or mini loaf pans and freeze leftovers for use on another day. Enjoy leftover meat loaf on slices of soft bread for a hearty meat loaf sandwich.

¾ cup quick-cooking oats	2 large eggs, beaten
½ cup milk	2 teaspoons Worcestershire sauce
1 medium-size onion, peeled	¼ cup ketchup
2 pounds ground turkey breast	½ teaspoon salt
½ cup seeded and chopped red bell pepper	Freshly ground black pepper
	1 (8-ounce) can tomato sauce

1. Preheat the oven to 350°F.
2. In a small bowl, stir together the oats and milk. Thinly slice one quarter of the onion and set aside. Finely chop the remaining onion. In a large bowl, combine the turkey, oat mixture, chopped onion, bell pepper, eggs, Worcestershire sauce, ketchup, salt, and a few grinds of black pepper. Mix just until well combined.
3. Transfer the mixture to a 9 by 9-inch baking dish or a standard loaf pan and shape into a loaf about 5 inches wide and 2½ inches high. Pour the tomato sauce over the meat loaf and sprinkle with the sliced onion. Bake for about 1 hour, or until an instant-read thermometer inserted into the center registers 160°F.
4. Remove from the oven and let rest for 10 to 15 minutes before slicing.

Nutritional Analysis: Calories 243, Total Fat 11 g, Saturated Fat 3 g, Cholesterol 133 mg, Sodium 467 mg, Carbohydrates 12 g, Dietary Fiber 2 g, Protein 26 g

Symptom	
Lack of Appetite	+
Nausea, Vomiting, or Heartburn	+
Constipation	+
Diarrhea	+
Fatigue	+
Mouth Sores	
Dry Mouth	+
Chewing or Swallowing Difficulty	+
Taste Aversion— Sweet	+
Taste Aversion— Sour & Bitter	+
Lack of Taste	+
Smells Bother	+

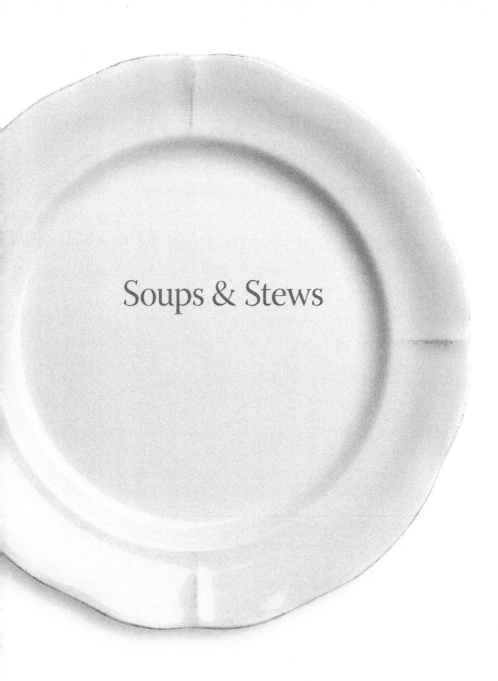

Soups & Stews

Cool Cucumber Avocado Soup ①

Time: Prep: 15 minutes
Serves 4

This soup is cold and creamy and is great for someone with difficulty chewing or swallowing. Want to add a little more tang? Try using buttermilk instead of regular milk. If you have mouth sores, nausea, or heartburn, avoid the tomato topping. Use leftover soup like a salad dressing or salsa, drizzling it over greens or roasted vegetables, or add it to sandwiches or tacos.

2 avocados, peeled and pitted

½ medium-size cucumber, peeled and cut into smaller pieces

1 cup cold water

½ cup milk

2 to 4 tablespoons freshly squeezed lemon juice

2 ice cubes

½ teaspoon salt, plus more to taste (optional)

Toppings

½ cup chopped tomatoes

2 teaspoons olive oil

Chopped fresh chives

3 sprigs fresh dill

1. Place the avocado, cucumber, water, milk, 2 tablespoons of the lemon juice, and the ice cubes and salt in a food processor or blender. Blend until completely smooth. Season to taste with more lemon juice or salt.
2. Top with the chopped tomatoes, a splash of olive oil, chopped chives, and some dill. For an extra kick, add your favorite hot sauce.

Nutritional Analysis (does not include toppings): Calories 178, Total Fat 15 g, Saturated Fat 2 g, Cholesterol 2 mg, Sodium 261 mg, Carbohydrates 11 g, Dietary Fiber 7 g, Protein 3 g

Nutritional Analysis (includes toppings): Calories 202, Total Fat 17 g, Saturated Fat 2 g, Cholesterol 2 mg, Sodium 262 mg, Carbohydrates 12 g, Dietary Fiber 7 g, Protein 3 g

Lack of Appetite	+
Nausea, Vomiting, or Heartburn	+
Constipation	+
Diarrhea	+
Fatigue	+
Mouth Sores	+
Dry Mouth	+
Chewing or Swallowing Difficulty	+
Taste Aversion—Sweet	+
Taste Aversion—Sour & Bitter	+
Lack of Taste	+
Smells Bother	+

Fruit Lovers' Gazpacho ①

Time: 30 minutes
Serves 4

This cold soup gets amped up by the addition of watermelon and bell pepper, and the combination of ginger, lime juice, and chili really wakes up the taste buds. Use leftover gazpacho just like a salsa and enjoy as a dip for cut-up vegetables or tortilla chips, or alongside Mexican dishes. Or freeze the soup into Popsicles for a soothing sweet and savory treat to relieve a dry mouth.

3 cups seeded and diced watermelon

1 celery rib, chopped

2 medium-size tomatoes, roughly chopped

½ medium-size cucumber, peeled and roughly chopped

1 medium-size yellow or orange bell pepper, seeded and roughly chopped

1 (1-inch) piece fresh ginger, peeled and minced

½ jalapeño or serrano pepper (optional if mouth sores)

Juice of 1 lime

Handful of fresh basil

Salt and freshly ground black pepper

1. Set aside five or six chunks of the watermelon and a couple of celery pieces for garnish.
2. Place the rest of the watermelon and celery in a blender or a food processor together with all the other ingredients, except the salt and black pepper. Pulse it until it develops a souplike consistency, taste, and season as desired.
3. Pour the soup into a container and place in the refrigerator to chill for at least 30 minutes to let the flavors develop.
4. When ready to serve, ladle the soup into bowls and top each bowl with the reserved watermelon and celery garnishes.

Nutritional Analysis: Calories 57, Total Fat 0 g, Saturated Fat 0 g, Cholesterol 0 mg, Sodium 12 mg, Carbohydrates 14 g, Dietary Fiber 2 g, Protein 2 g

♥ Nutritionist's Favorite to Savor
This recipe is my favorite because people do not normally think of fruit as being compatible with a soup! Such an easy way to enjoy colorful fruits and veggies with a touch of ginger to help manage nausea.

Lack of Appetite

Nausea, Vomiting, or Heartburn

Constipation

Diarrhea

Fatigue

Mouth Sores

Dry Mouth

Chewing or Swallowing Difficulty

Taste Aversion— Sweet

Taste Aversion— Sour & Bitter

Lack of Taste

Smells Bother

Great Greens Spinach and Kale Soup

Time: Prep: 15 minutes; Cook: 30 minutes
Serves 4

Time to get cozy with this warming wintry soup. There's double the greens for double the fun and a great helping of nutrients. Add cooked grains—quinoa, rice, kasha, or couscous—to the soup to bulk it up the next day.

1 tablespoon olive oil
1 medium-size onion, finely chopped
4 garlic cloves, finely chopped
Pinch of dried red pepper flakes
   (optional)
2 cups chopped fresh or thawed
   frozen spinach
2 cups chopped fresh or thawed

frozen kale
½ teaspoon ground nutmeg
4 cups water or low-sodium vegetable
   stock
1½ cups cooked white beans, or
   1 (15-ounce) can, drained and rinsed
Salt and freshly ground black pepper

1. Heat the olive oil in a large saucepan. Add the onion, garlic, and red pepper flakes and cook until slightly softened and the garlic and onions are translucent.
2. Stir in the spinach, kale, and nutmeg and gently cook for 1 minute. Add the water and white beans. Bring to a boil, lower the heat to low, and simmer for 20 more minutes. Season with salt and pepper to taste.
3. Serve as it is or blend until silky smooth. Both ways are delicious.

Nutritional Analysis: Calories 176, Total Fat 4 g, Saturated Fat 1 g, Cholesterol 0 mg, Sodium 178 mg, Carbohydrates 28 g, Dietary Fiber 7 g, Protein 9 g

Lack of Appetite	+
Nausea, Vomiting, or Heartburn	+
Constipation	+
Diarrhea	
Fatigue	+
Mouth Sores	+
Dry Mouth	+
Chewing or Swallowing Difficulty	+
Taste Aversion— Sweet	+
Taste Aversion— Sour & Bitter	+
Lack of Taste	+
Smells Bother	+

Tuscan White Bean Vegetable Stew

Time: Prep: 15 minutes; Cook: 45 minutes
Serves 6

Pureeing some of the beans and stirring in torn pieces of bread turn this dish from a soup into a hearty wholesome stew. Finish the stew with some lemon zest to brighten the flavors. This soup combines all of the food groups and serves as a great one-pot meal for times when you are experiencing fatigue and lack of appetite.

1 tablespoon olive oil	1 bunch kale, stemmed and chopped
2 celery ribs, chopped	1½ cups cooked white beans,
2 garlic cloves, chopped	or 1 (15-ounce) can, drained
1 medium-size carrot, chopped	and rinsed
1½ cups peeled, seeded, and chopped	4 ounces bread, crusts removed,
butternut squash	torn into bite-size pieces
½ medium-size red onion, chopped	Salt and freshly ground black pepper
1 (14-ounce) can crushed tomatoes	Zest and juice of 1 lemon

1. Heat the olive oil in a large pot over medium heat, then add the celery, garlic, carrot, squash, and red onion. Cook for 10 to 15 minutes, so the vegetables sweat.
2. Stir in the tomatoes and simmer for another 5 minutes, until the mixture thickens slightly.
3. Add the kale, 1 cup of the beans, and 4 cups of water. Bring to a boil.
4. While the soup comes to a boil, remove ½ cup of the simmering soup liquid, add the remaining ½ cup of white beans to it, and puree.
5. Stir the bean puree and bread pieces into the soup. Simmer, stirring occasionally, until the bread breaks down and the soup thickens, for about 15 minutes. Add salt and pepper to taste. Add the lemon zest and juice.

Nutritional Analysis: Calories 293, Total Fat 6 g, Saturated Fat 1 g, Cholesterol 17 mg, Sodium 393 mg, Carbohydrates 51 g, Dietary Fiber 10 g, Protein 13 g

Sidebar (left margin):
- + Lack of Appetite
- + Nausea, Vomiting, or Heartburn
- + Constipation
- + Diarrhea
- + Fatigue
- + Mouth Sores
- + Dry Mouth
- + Chewing or Swallowing Difficulty
- + Taste Aversion—Sweet
- + Taste Aversion—Sour & Bitter
- + Lack of Taste
- + Smells Bother

Hearty Tomato Lentil Soup

Time: Prep: 15 minutes; Cook: 30 minutes
Serves 6

Cook up a large pot of this soup and enjoy it for a light lunch all week long. Cumin, coriander, ginger, cinnamon, and turmeric add healing warmth. Try pureeing leftover soup and enjoying it as a sauce or dip for vegetables or bread.

2 tablespoons olive oil

1 medium-size onion, chopped

2 garlic cloves, minced

1 teaspoon ground cumin

1 teaspoon ground coriander

1 teaspoon grated fresh ginger

¼ teaspoon ground cinnamon

1 teaspoon ground turmeric

⅛ teaspoon freshly ground black
   pepper

2 medium-size carrots, chopped

1 medium-size sweet potato,
   chopped

2 celery ribs, chopped

1 cup dried brown or green lentils

4 cups vegetable stock or water

1 (15-ounce) can diced tomatoes

1 teaspoon salt

¼ cup chopped fresh cilantro
   (optional)

1. Heat the olive oil in a large pot over medium heat. Add the onion and garlic and sauté until soft. Add the cumin, coriander, ginger, cinnamon, turmeric, and pepper and sauté for a few more minutes. Add the carrots, sweet potato, celery, lentils, stock, and tomatoes. Stir softly and bring to a low boil. Lower the heat to a simmer, cover, and cook for 45 minutes, or until the lentils and potato are tender.

2. Stir in the salt. Serve the stew garnished with cilantro, if using.

Nutritional Analysis: Calories 206, Total Fat 5 g, Saturated Fat 1 g, Cholesterol 0 mg, Sodium 596 mg, Carbohydrates 32 g, Dietary Fiber 8 g, Protein 8 g

Lack of Appetite	+
Nausea, Vomiting, or Heartburn	
Constipation	+
Diarrhea	+
Fatigue	+
Mouth Sores	
Dry Mouth	+
Chewing or Swallowing Difficulty	+
Taste Aversion— Sweet	+
Taste Aversion— Sour & Bitter	+
Lack of Taste	+
Smells Bother	+

Orzo Kale Soup

Time: Prep: 15 minutes; Cook: 30 minutes
Serves 4

Lack of Appetite

Nausea, Vomiting, or Heartburn

Constipation

Diarrhea

Fatigue

Mouth Sores

Dry Mouth

Chewing or Swallowing Difficulty

Taste Aversion— Sweet

Taste Aversion— Sour & Bitter

Lack of Taste

Smells Bother

Orzo is a petite pasta that works great in soups. Toss in cooked shredded chicken or turkey to bulk up the soup. Reduce or omit the tomatoes if you need to reduce the acidity.

2 tablespoons olive oil

1 medium-size onion, chopped

2 medium-size carrots, peeled and chopped

2 garlic cloves, minced

1 (15-ounce) can diced tomatoes

2 cups vegetable stock

1½ cups cooked white beans, or 1 (15-ounce) can, drained and rinsed

½ cup whole wheat orzo

4 cups chopped kale

Salt and freshly ground black pepper

¼ cup freshly grated Parmesan cheese (optional)

1. Heat the olive oil in a large pot over medium heat. Add the onion and carrots and sauté for about 5 minutes, or until the veggies are beginning to soften. Add the garlic and sauté for 1 minute more.
2. Add the tomatoes, stock, and white beans. Bring to a boil, then lower the heat to a simmer. Cover and cook for about 15 minutes.
3. Add the orzo and simmer the soup for about 10 more minutes, or until the orzo becomes tender. Add the kale and cook for 1 to 2 minutes more, or until the kale is tender. Season to taste with salt and pepper.
4. To serve, ladle a generous portion of soup into each bowl. Top with freshly grated Parmesan, if using.

Nutritional Analysis (without the Parmesan): Calories 287, Total Fat 8 g, Saturated Fat 1 g, Cholesterol 0 mg, Sodium 333 mg, Carbohydrates 45 g, Dietary Fiber 10 g, Protein 13 g

Nutritional Analysis (with 1 tablespoon Parmesan): Calories 308, Total Fat 8 g, Saturated Fat 2 g, Cholesterol 4 mg, Sodium 423 mg, Carbohydrates 46 g, Dietary Fiber 10 g, Protein 14 g

Carrot Ginger Soup with Cashew Cream

Time: Prep: 15 minutes; Cook: 30 minutes
Serves 4

Pureed carrot soup begs for a swirl of something creamy, and using cashew cream adds richness without weighing you down. Add some texture to leftover soup—a handful of chickpeas, cubed tofu, or cooked brown rice are all great additions.

1 tablespoon olive oil
1 medium-size onion, diced
½ cup diced celery
1 (1-inch) piece fresh ginger, grated
4 cups vegetable stock
1 medium-size russet potato, cut into

large pieces
1¼ pounds carrots, chopped
  (about 8 carrots)
Salt (2 generous pinches to start)
1¼ teaspoons ground nutmeg
⅔ cup Cashew Cream (page 222)

1. Heat the olive oil in a medium-size pot and sauté the onion, celery, and ginger until the onion is translucent, for about 10 minutes.
2. Add the stock, potato, carrots, salt, and nutmeg to the pot. Bring the liquid to a boil, and then lower the heat to a simmer. Simmer for about 20 minutes, or until the carrots and potato are tender.
3. When the carrots are tender, remove from the heat. Puree the soup in batches in a blender, or use an immersion blender.
4. Transfer the blended soup back to the pot, and warm through. Stir in ⅓ cup of the cashew cream. To serve the soup, ladle into bowls and top with a swirl of additional cashew cream.

Nutritional Analysis (does not include Cashew Cream): Calories 162, Total Fat 4 g, Saturated Fat 1 g, Cholesterol 0 mg, Sodium 372 mg, Carbohydrates 30 g, Dietary Fiber 6 g, Protein 3 g

Nutritional Analysis (includes Cashew Cream): Calories 215, Total Fat 8 g, Saturated Fat 2 g, Cholesterol 0 mg, Sodium 373 mg, Carbohydrates 33 g, Dietary Fiber 6 g, Protein 4 g

Nutritionist's Favorite to Savor
This recipe is my favorite because it is a wonderfully warm soup that, if made in bulk, freezes really well for future use. Swirling in cashew cream amps up the heartiness of the soup.

Lack of Appetite	+
Nausea, Vomiting, or Heartburn	+
Constipation	+
Diarrhea	+
Fatigue	+
Mouth Sores	+
Dry Mouth	+
Chewing or Swallowing Difficulty	+
Taste Aversion—Sweet	+
Taste Aversion—Sour & Bitter	+
Lack of Taste	+
Smells Bother	+

Simple Mushroom Soup

Time: Prep: 15 minutes; Cook: 30 minutes
Serves 2

+	Lack of Appetite
+	Nausea, Vomiting, or Heartburn
+	Constipation
+	Diarrhea
+	Fatigue
+	Mouth Sores
+	Dry Mouth
+	Chewing or Swallowing Difficulty
+	Taste Aversion— Sweet
+	Taste Aversion— Sour & Bitter
+	Lack of Taste
+	Smells Bother

Cremini mushrooms are very versatile and can be found in most grocery stores and farmers' markets. Want to branch out? Swap out some of the cremini mushrooms for a bolder wild mushroom variety, such as shiitake, maitake, or wood ear. Spruce up leftover soup by adding some Cashew Cream (page 222); fresh herbs, such as thyme or rosemary; or a drizzle of sesame oil. Leftover soup also works as a rich sauce for chicken or tofu.

1 tablespoon olive oil or unsalted butter

8 ounces cremini mushrooms, sliced

½ small onion, chopped

1½ cups vegetable stock

Salt and freshly ground black pepper

1. Heat the oil in a large pot over medium-high heat. Add the mushrooms and onion and cook for 5 to 8 minutes, or until the mushrooms turn from gray to golden and most of the liquid they release has evaporated.
2. Add the vegetable stock and bring the soup to a boil. Lower the heat and simmer for 5 to 10 minutes. Add salt and pepper to taste.
3. Enjoy the soup as is or puree some or all of the soup for a thicker texture.

Nutritional Analysis: Calories 103, Total Fat 7 g, Saturated Fat 1 g, Cholesterol 0 mg, Sodium 233 mg, Carbohydrates 9 g, Dietary Fiber 2 g, Protein 3 g

Asparagus Potato Curry

Time: Prep: 15 minutes; Cook: 30 minutes
Serves 4 to 6

Curry is a great addition to your flavor arsenal to help wake up the taste buds. Plain yogurt gets stirred in at the last minute to add a nice cooling contrast to the spices. Enjoy this as a side dish or as a complete meal by mixing in a protein of choice and enjoying over a bed of rice.

4 medium-size potatoes (any variety), cut into ½-inch cubes

2 cups chopped asparagus

2 tablespoons olive oil

1 large red onion, diced

3 garlic cloves, minced

1 tablespoon minced fresh ginger

1 tablespoon ground coriander

¾ teaspoon ground cumin

¾ teaspoon ground turmeric

½ teaspoon chili powder

1 cup plain yogurt

¼ cup minced fresh cilantro

2 tablespoons freshly squeezed lemon juice

1. Place a few inches of water in a lidded pot fitted with a steamer basket. Bring the water to a simmer over medium heat. Place the potatoes in the steamer, place the lid on the pot, and steam for 15 minutes, or until tender. Add the asparagus and steam for another 5 to 10 minutes, or until both the potatoes and asparagus are tender. Remove from the steamer and set aside.
2. Heat the olive oil in a large skillet over medium heat. Sauté the onion, garlic, and ginger for 5 minutes, or until tender. Add the coriander, cumin, turmeric, and chili powder. Cook for 2 minutes, stirring frequently.
3. Lower the heat to low and add the potatoes and asparagus. Toss well to coat with the spices. Cover and heat for 2 to 3 minutes.
4. Remove from the heat and let cool slightly. Slowly mix in the yogurt. Sprinkle with the fresh cilantro and lemon juice.

Nutritional Analysis: Calories 306, Total Fat 8 g, Saturated Fat 2 g, Cholesterol 4 mg, Sodium 65 mg, Carbohydrates 51 g, Dietary Fiber g, Protein 10 g

Lack of Appetite	+
Nausea, Vomiting, or Heartburn	
Constipation	+
Diarrhea	
Fatigue	+
Mouth Sores	
Dry Mouth	+
Chewing or Swallowing Difficulty	+
Taste Aversion— Sweet	+
Taste Aversion— Sour & Bitter	+
Lack of Taste	+
Smells Bother	+

Spiced and Simmered Green Lentils

Time: Prep: 15 minutes; Cook: 45 minutes
Serves 4 to 6

Lack of
Appetite

Nausea,
Vomiting, or
Heartburn

Constipation

Diarrhea

Fatigue

Mouth
Sores

Dry
Mouth

Chewing or
Swallowing
Difficulty

Taste
Aversion—
Sweet

Taste
Aversion—
Sour & Bitter

Lack of
Taste

Smells
Bother

Cloves add a unique subtle flavor to these green lentils. Add a squeeze of lime if experiencing lack of taste or metallic taste. For an extra-special variation, roast a head of garlic and squeeze the roasted cloves into the soup at the very end of cooking. To roast garlic, slice the top off a head of garlic, drizzle with olive oil and salt, and wrap in foil. Place in a 375°F oven for about 40 minutes, or until the cloves can be easily squeezed out of the casing.

1 cup dried green lentils

1 tablespoon olive oil, plus
    more for drizzling

¼ teaspoon ground cloves

1 small onion, chopped

1 medium-size carrot, chopped

1 celery rib, trimmed and chopped

1 garlic clove, smashed

1 bay leaf

3½ cups Aromatic Vegetable Stock
    (page 216)

Salt and freshly ground black pepper

1 scallion, finely chopped, for garnish

1. Rinse the lentils in a strainer under cold running water. Put the lentils in a medium-size saucepan, cover with cold water, and bring to a boil.
2. Cook for 2 minutes, then pour out the lentils through a strainer. Drain, then rinse the lentils again. Set aside.
3. Heat the olive oil in a large pot over medium-high heat. Add the cloves, onion, carrot, celery, and garlic. Sauté for about 5 minutes.
4. Add the bay leaf and vegetable stock, stir in the lentils, and bring to a boil.
5. Lower the heat to a steady simmer, cover, and cook for 30 minutes, or until the lentils are tender. Season with salt and pepper to taste.
6. Add the chopped scallion and finish with a drizzle of olive oil.

Nutritional Analysis: Calories 191, Total Fat 2 g, Saturated Fat 0 g, Cholesterol 0 mg, Sodium 148 mg, Carbohydrates 34 g, Dietary Fiber 9 g, Protein 11 g

Sweet Potatoes with Red Lentils and Coconut

Time: Prep: 15 minutes; Cook: 45 minutes
Serves 6 to 8

Red lentils break down during cooking, almost melting into the stew. The buttery flesh of the sweet potato can hold the flavor of the coconut milk well. Experiment with different spices to help enhance flavor and combat taste aversion. Reduce the spices as needed to adjust to flavor preference. To make the sweet potatoes easier to chop, poke holes in the sweet potatoes with a fork and heat in a microwave on high power for 5 minutes. Let cool for 2 minutes, then chop.

3 large sweet potatoes, peeled and
    diced (about 6 cups)
3 cups vegetable stock
1 medium-size yellow onion,
    chopped
4 garlic cloves, minced

2 teaspoons ground coriander
2 teaspoons garam masala
2 teaspoons chili powder
½ teaspoon salt
1½ cups dried red lentils
1 (15-ounce) can coconut milk

1. Place the sweet potatoes, vegetable stock, onion, garlic, spices, and salt in a large pot. Bring to a boil.
2. Add the lentils and stir once. Stir in the coconut milk and 1 cup of water. Lower the heat to low, cover, and simmer for 30 to 50 minutes, or until the lentils absorb most of the liquid and are soft.

Nutritional Analysis: Calories 371, Total Fat 15 g, Saturated Fat 12 g, Cholesterol 0 mg, Sodium 295 mg, Carbohydrates 47 g, Dietary Fiber 10 g, Protein 16 g

Lack of Appetite	+
Nausea, Vomiting, or Heartburn	+
Constipation	+
Diarrhea	+
Fatigue	+
Mouth Sores	+
Dry Mouth	+
Chewing or Swallowing Difficulty	+
Taste Aversion— Sweet	+
Taste Aversion— Sour & Bitter	+
Lack of Taste	+
Smells Bother	+

Veggie Loaded 3-Bean Chili

Time: Prep: 15 minutes; Cook: 30 minutes
Serves 8

The contrasting textures of the three types of beans adds a chew to the chili. Swap out one type of bean for some cooked lean ground turkey or chicken, for extra protein. This chili is begging to be served with a thick square of warm corn bread!

1 tablespoon olive oil

1 small onion, chopped

1 medium-size red bell pepper, seeded and chopped

1 jalapeño pepper, seeded and chopped (optional)

1 medium-size carrot, chopped

1 medium-size zucchini, chopped

3 garlic cloves

1 (15-ounce) can kidney beans, drained

and rinsed

1 (15-ounce) can black beans, drained and rinsed

1 (15-ounce) can chickpeas, drained and rinsed

1 (28-ounce) can diced tomatoes

1 tablespoon dried oregano

1 tablespoon chili powder

1 cup water or vegetable stock

Salt and freshly ground black pepper

1. Heat the olive oil in a large pot over medium heat. Add the onion, bell pepper, jalapeño, if using, carrot, and zucchini and cook until the vegetables just start to become tender, for about 5 minutes.
2. Add the garlic, beans, tomatoes, oregano, chili powder, and water. Stir.
3. Bring to a boil, stirring occasionally to combine all the flavors. Once boiling, cover the pot and lower the heat to a simmer. Simmer for 30 minutes, stirring occasionally to prevent sticking.
4. Add salt and black pepper to taste. Ladle into bowls and eat.

Nutritional Analysis: Calories 179, Total Fat 3 g, Saturated Fat 1 g, Cholesterol 0 mg, Sodium 482 mg, Carbohydrates 29 g, Dietary Fiber 7 g, Protein 9 g

Stretch and Save: Make "loaded baked potatoes" with leftover chili. Poke holes into russet or sweet potatoes and roast in the oven at 400°F for 1 hour (or cook in a microwave on a high power setting for 5 to 7 minutes) or until soft. Slit the potatoes lengthwise and top with the chili.

Lack of Appetite

Nausea, Vomiting, or Heartburn

Constipation

Diarrhea

Fatigue

Mouth Sores

Dry Mouth

Chewing or Swallowing Difficulty

Taste Aversion— Sweet

Taste Aversion— Sour & Bitter

Lack of Taste

Smells Bother

Sweet Potato Black Bean Chili

Time: Prep: 15 minutes; Cook: 30 minutes
Serves 6

If you have the time, try making this chili using ½ pound of dried black beans instead of canned beans. The beans should be soaked overnight, drained, and then placed in a pot with water to cover by a few inches. Bring to a boil, lower the heat to low, and simmer for 1½ to 3 hours, or until the beans are soft but not falling apart. Add to the chili in the same manner as you would the canned beans.

1 tablespoon olive oil

½ medium-size yellow onion, chopped

2 garlic cloves, smashed

2 teaspoons ground cumin

¼ teaspoon ground cinnamon

1 teaspoon chili powder

1 medium-size sweet potato, peeled and diced into 1-inch cubes

2 cups Aromatic Vegetable Stock (page 216)

2 (15-ounce) cans black beans, drained and rinsed (see headnote)

1 tablespoon tomato paste

Salt

Chopped fresh cilantro, to finish

Hot sauce, to finish

1. Heat the olive oil in a large stockpot over medium-high heat. Add the onion and sauté for 5 minutes, or until translucent. Add the garlic, cumin, cinnamon, and chili powder and sauté for 1 minute more.

2. Add the sweet potato, stock, black beans, and tomato paste. Bring to a boil. Simmer for about 10 minutes. Remove from the heat, add salt to taste, cilantro, and hot sauce to taste.

Nutritional Analysis: Calories 169, Total Fat 3 g, Saturated Fat 0 g, Cholesterol 0 mg, Sodium 237 mg, Carbohydrates 28 g, Dietary Fiber 9 g, Protein 8 g

Lack of Appetite	+
Nausea, Vomiting, or Heartburn	+
Constipation	+
Diarrhea	+
Fatigue	+
Mouth Sores	
Dry Mouth	+
Chewing or Swallowing Difficulty	+
Taste Aversion— Sweet	+
Taste Aversion— Sour & Bitter	+
Lack of Taste	+
Smells Bother	+

Vegetable Chicken Soup

Time: Prep: 15 minutes; Cook: 30 minutes
Serves 6

+	Lack of Appetite
+	Nausea, Vomiting, or Heartburn
+	Constipation
+	Diarrhea
+	Fatigue
+	Mouth Sores
+	Dry Mouth
+	Chewing or Swallowing Difficulty
	Taste Aversion— Sweet
+	Taste Aversion— Sour & Bitter
+	Lack of Taste
+	Smells Bother

As the number one comfort food, chicken soup is extremely versatile and can work well for most symptoms. Add your favorite mini pasta or grain for an even heartier meal. Even the broth itself can be soothing to a sore mouth or stomach.

1 chicken, cut into parts
6 carrots, chopped
4 celery ribs, chopped
2 medium-size white onions, halved
½ garlic head, sliced
2 bay leaves

4 whole peppercorns
Salt
1 bunch of spinach or chard, chopped
Handful of chopped fresh parsley, thyme, or dill

1. Place the chicken, two thirds of the carrots, and the celery, onions, garlic, bay leaves, peppercorns, and a pinch of salt in a large pot. Fill the pot with cold water to cover, then bring to a boil over high heat.
2. Lower the heat to a simmer and cook for 1 hour, skimming off the fat from time to time.
3. After 1 hour, drain the stock into a separate pot. Discard the vegetables. Let the chicken cool, then chop the meat into bite-size pieces.
4. Add the chicken pieces, remaining chopped carrot, and greens to the stock. Place over medium heat and simmer for 20 to 30 minutes.
5. Serve and garnish with your choice of herb.

Nutritional Analysis: Calories 162, Total Fat 4 g, Saturated Fat 1 g, Cholesterol 77 mg, Sodium 171 mg, Carbohydrates 7 g, Dietary Fiber 2 g, Protein 25 g

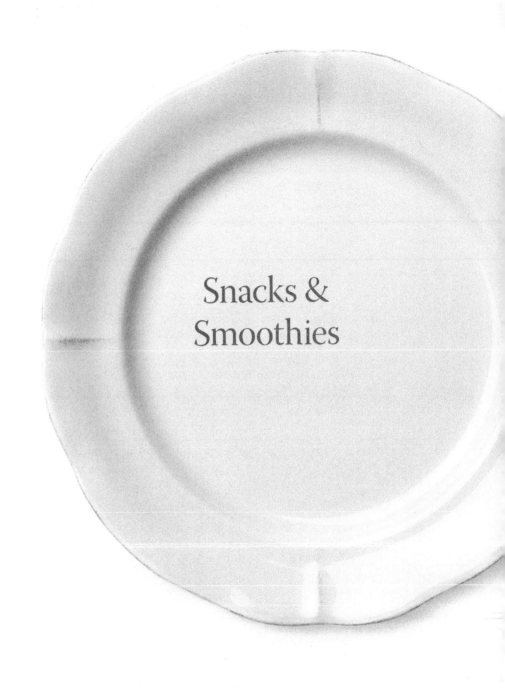

Snacks &
Smoothies

Baked Parmesan Swiss Chard Chips Ⓘ

Time: Prep: 5 minutes; Cook: 15 minutes
Serves 2

Kale works great for this recipe as well. For a vegan option, try a few shakes of nutritional yeast instead of Parmesan, for a cheesy flavor. Crumble left-over "chips" into a fine powder and shake it over the popcorn to make a green popcorn snack!

1 bunch Swiss chard	Sprinkle of salt
1 teaspoon olive oil	½ cup shredded Parmesan cheese

1. Preheat the oven to 350°F.
2. Wash and thoroughly dry the chard. Remove and discard the leaves from the thick stems and tear the leaves into bite-size pieces.
3. Place the leaves on a baking sheet and rub them with the olive oil. Arrange in an even layer and sprinkle with salt. Place the baking sheet in the oven.
4. After 12 to 15 minutes of baking, toss and mix the chard to ensure that the leaves crisp evenly. Add the shredded Parmesan cheese, and place back in the oven to bake for an additional 5 minutes. Keep a close eye on the chips so they do not burn. Remove the chips from the oven once crisp.

Nutritional Analysis: Calories 133, Total Fat 8 g, Saturated Fat 4 g, Cholesterol 14 mg, Sodium 701 mg, Carbohydrates 7 g, Dietary Fiber 2 g, Protein 10 g

Nutritionist's Favorite to Savor
This recipe is my favorite because while many people are intimidated by Swiss chard, this easy snack simply requires tearing the leaves and baking in the oven. You will get hooked on this nutrient-rich vegetable in no time.

Sidebar

- + Lack of Appetite
- + Nausea, Vomiting, or Heartburn
- + Constipation
- Diarrhea
- + Fatigue
- Mouth Sores
- + Dry Mouth
- Chewing or Swallowing Difficulty
- + Taste Aversion— Sweet
- + Taste Aversion— Sour & Bitter
- + Lack of Taste
- + Smells Bother

Cinnamon Pear Chips

Time: Prep: 15 minutes; Cook: 1 hour
Makes 30 chips

This is a perfect snack to munch on for added fiber and a simple, easy way to add more fruits when symptoms may get in the way. Don't have pears? This works great with apples, too.

2 medium-size crisp pears, washed and dried

½ teaspoon ground cinnamon

1. Preheat the oven to 275°F. Line two baking sheets with parchment paper or silicone mats.
2. Core the pears. Using a mandoline, cut the pears into 1/16-inch-thick slices. Or slice the pears thinly by hand. Arrange the pear slices on the prepared baking sheets.
3. Sprinkle the cinnamon over the pear slices. Bake the pears until almost dry, about 1 hour, rotating the baking sheets halfway through to ensure even baking.
4. Cool the pear chips and serve, or store in an airtight container for up to 2 days.

Nutritional Analysis (per 15 chips): Calories 113, Total Fat 0 g, Saturated Fat 0 g, Cholesterol 0 mg, Sodium 2 mg, Carbohydrates 27 g, Dietary Fiber 6 g, Protein 1 g

Lack of Appetite	+
Nausea, Vomiting, or Heartburn	+
Constipation	+
Diarrhea	+
Fatigue	+
Mouth Sores	+
Dry Mouth	+
Chewing or Swallowing Difficulty	
Taste Aversion— Sweet	+
Taste Aversion— Sour & Bitter	+
Lack of Taste	+
Smells Bother	+

Cranberry Date Chocolate Granola Bites ⓘ

Time: 30 minutes
Makes 12 to 15 bites

These bites are a great snack to make ahead and take with you on the go. Leftover bites will keep in the freezer for up to a month.

Lack of
Appetite

Nausea,
Vomiting, or
Heartburn

Constipation

Diarrhea

Fatigue

Mouth
Sores

Dry
Mouth

Chewing or
Swallowing
Difficulty

Taste
Aversion—
Sweet

Taste
Aversion—
Sour & Bitter

Lack of
Taste

Smells
Bother

1¼ cups quick or rolled oats
¼ cup dried cranberries
¼ cup chopped walnuts
¼ cup large coconut flakes or unsweetened shredded coconut
2 tablespoons mini dark chocolate chips or cacao nibs

2 tablespoons pitted and chopped Medjool dates
3 tablespoons honey
2 tablespoons almond butter
2 tablespoons coconut oil or unsalted butter
¼ teaspoon salt
¼ teaspoon ground cinnamon

1. In a bowl, combine the oats, cranberries, walnuts, coconut, chocolate chips, and chopped dates and set aside.
2. In a medium-size pot, combine the honey, almond butter, coconut oil, salt, and cinnamon. Heat over medium-low heat, stirring constantly, until the mixture is hot. Pour in the dry ingredients, turn off the heat, and stir thoroughly to combine everything. You may need to add 1 to 2 tablespoons of water if the mixture looks dry. Set aside to cool to room temperature, for 15 to 30 minutes.
3. Form the mixture into balls the size of a Ping-Pong ball. Press each ball together very firmly to help hold the shape. Store in the refrigerator.

Nutritional Analysis: Calories 125, Total Fat 7 g, Saturated Fat 3 g, Cholesterol 0 mg, Sodium 38 mg, Carbohydrates 15 g, Dietary Fiber 2 g, Protein 2 g

Roasted Applesauce

Time: Prep: 15 minutes; Cook: 30 minutes
Serves 8 (makes 4 cups applesauce)

Applesauce tastes great swirled into oatmeal, cottage cheese, or yogurt for a cozy breakfast or snack. It also pairs well with savory foods, such as cheese and crackers, and poultry. It is also a versatile snack that is easy tolerated with any digestion-related symptom.

Nonstick cooking spray
8 to 10 baking apples, such as
   Granny Smith, McIntosh, or
   Pink Lady (3 pounds), peeled,
   cut in half, and cored

¼ cup light or dark brown sugar
¼ teaspoon ground cinnamon,
   or to taste
Pinch of salt

1. Preheat the oven to 375°F. Prepare a rimmed baking sheet with a light layer of cooking spray.
2. Place the apple halves, cut side down, on the baking sheet and cover tightly with foil.
3. Bake the apples for 30 to 40 minutes, or until tender. Set aside to cool.
4. Combine the apples, brown sugar, cinnamon, and salt in a food processor (or mash by hand) and mix until pureed. Add up to 3 table-spoons of water, if necessary, to thin.
5. Enjoy warm, at room temperature, or cold.

Nutritional Analysis: Calories 99, Total Fat 0 g, Saturated Fat 0 g, Cholesterol 0 mg, Sodium 9 mg, Carbohydrates 26 g, Dietary Fiber 2 g, Protein 0 g

Stretch and Save: In the mood to bake? Replace half of the butter or oil in a recipe with applesauce, for a lower-fat baked good.

Symptom	
Lack of Appetite	+
Nausea, Vomiting, or Heartburn	+
Constipation	+
Diarrhea	+
Fatigue	+
Mouth Sores	+
Dry Mouth	+
Chewing or Swallowing Difficulty	+
Taste Aversion— Sweet	
Taste Aversion— Sour & Bitter	+
Lack of Taste	+
Smells Bother	+

Whole Wheat Chocolate Raisin Zucchini Bread

Time: Prep: 15 minutes; Cook: 50 minutes
Serves 10

Lack of
Appetite

Nausea,
Vomiting, or
Heartburn

Constipation

Diarrhea

Fatigue

Mouth
Sores

Dry
Mouth

Chewing or
Swallowing
Difficulty

Taste
Aversion—
Sweet

Taste
Aversion—
Sour & Bitter

Lack of
Taste

Smells
Bother

Zucchini and chocolate are a wonderful flavor combination and a great way to enhance the vegetable component of this recipe. Grating the zucchini on the small holes of a box grater helps the small tufts blend right into the bread. Leftover zucchini bread can be frozen and kept for up to a month. Wrap individual slices in plastic wrap, for easy thawing.

⅔ cup vegetable oil

2 large eggs

1 cup sugar

1½ cups whole wheat flour

¾ teaspoon baking soda

½ teaspoon salt

1 teaspoon ground cinnamon

½ teaspoon ground nutmeg

2 cups grated zucchini (from 1 large
    or 2 small zucchini)

½ cup raisins

½ cup dark chocolate chips

1. Preheat the oven to 350°F. Grease a 9 by 5-inch loaf pan.
2. In a bowl, whisk together the vegetable oil and eggs.
3. In separate bowl, sift together the sugar, flour, baking soda, salt, cinnamon, and nutmeg. Mix in the egg mixture. Fold in the grated zucchini, raisins, and chocolate chips.
4. Pour into the prepared loaf pan. Bake for 50 minutes, or until a thin knife inserted into the center of the loaf comes out clean. Let cool on a wire rack for about 10 minutes.
5. After 10 minutes, run an offset spatula around the bread and invert it out of the loaf pan onto the wire rack. Let cool completely.
6. Slice and eat.

Nutritional Analysis: Calories 381, Total Fat 20 g, Saturated Fat 4 g, Cholesterol 43 mg, Sodium 211 mg, Carbohydrates 51 g, Dietary Fiber 4 g, Protein 5 g

Peaches and Cream Oat Smoothie

Time: 5 minutes
Serves 1

Sipping on a smoothie can help you get the nutrition your body needs. Peaches are in season during the summer months, but you can make this smoothie any time of year with frozen peaches. The rolled oats and flax-seeds in this drink add extra nutrition, making the smoothie feel like a meal. If you are experiencing bloating, omit the flaxseeds.

½ cup rolled oats

⅓ cup plain yogurt

¾ cup milk

1 small peach, pitted, or ½ cup frozen peaches

½ medium-size frozen or fresh banana, sliced

1 tablespoon ground flaxseeds

Pinch of salt

1. Combine all the ingredients in a blender.
2. Blend and pour into a large cup or bowl.

Nutritional Analysis: Calories 412, Total Fat 9 g, Saturated Fat 3 g, Cholesterol 14 mg, Sodium 138 mg, Carbohydrates 70 g, Dietary Fiber 9 g, Protein 19 g

Lack of Appetite	+
Nausea, Vomiting, or Heartburn	+
Constipation	+
Diarrhea	+
Fatigue	+
Mouth Sores	+
Dry Mouth	+
Chewing or Swallowing Difficulty	+
Taste Aversion—Sweet	
Taste Aversion—Sour & Bitter	+
Lack of Taste	+
Smells Bother	+

Avocado Mango Smoothie ①

Time: 5 minutes
Serves 2

With leafy greens, vitamin C–rich mangoes, and healthy fat from the avocado and tahini, this is a true "power smoothie." Make it ahead of time and freeze into Popsicles to soothe a dry mouth.

2 cups milk

4 cups leafy greens, such as spinach or kale, hard stems removed

1 avocado, peeled and pitted

1½ cups frozen mango cubes, slightly thawed

1 tablespoon tahini

1 tablespoon honey (optional)

1. Put the milk and leafy greens in a blender and blend until the greens are fully smooth and incorporated.
2. Add the avocado, mango, tahini, and honey, if using.
3. Pour into two glasses and enjoy.

Nutritional Analysis: Calories 418, Total Fat 21 g, Saturated Fat 4 g, Cholesterol 12 mg, Sodium 194 mg, Carbohydrates 52 g, Dietary Fiber 12 g, Protein 14 g

Nutritionist's Favorite to Savor
This recipe is my favorite because it includes a unique combination of ingredients—sesame paste, vitamin C–rich mangoes, and the heart-healthy fat of avocados. Smoothies are so helpful for cancer patients, for getting quick nutrition between meals or in use as a meal substitute.

Lack of
Appetite

Nausea,
Vomiting, or
Heartburn

Constipation

Diarrhea

Fatigue

Mouth
Sores

Dry
Mouth

Chewing or
Swallowing
Difficulty

Taste
Aversion—
Sweet

Taste
Aversion—
Sour & Bitter

Lack of
Taste

Smells
Bother

Blueberry Green Nut Butter Smoothie ⓘ

Time: 5 minutes
Serves 1

This is a great introduction to a green smoothie because the sweetness from the banana and dates and the creaminess from the peanut butter help mellow the flavor of the leafy greens. Green smoothies are especially good if you have a lack of appetite because they provide a lot of nutrition in just a few sips.

¾ cup frozen blueberries

1 cup leafy greens, such as spinach
   or kale

1 tablespoon peanut butter or
   any nut butter

¾ cup milk

½ medium-size frozen or
   fresh ripe banana, sliced

2 Medjool dates, pitted

½ cup ice

1. Place all the ingredients into a blender.
2. Blend until smooth. Pour into a glass and enjoy!

Nutritional Analysis: Calories 413, Total Fat 11 g, Saturated Fat 3 g, Cholesterol 9 mg, Sodium 203 mg, Carbohydrates 76 g, Dietary Fiber 11 g, Protein 13 g

Lack of Appetite +

Nausea, Vomiting, or Heartburn +

Constipation +

Diarrhea +

Fatigue +

Mouth Sores +

Dry Mouth +

Chewing or Swallowing Difficulty +

Taste Aversion— Sweet

Taste Aversion— Sour & Bitter +

Lack of Taste +

Smells Bother +

Sweet Banana Date Oat Shake ◯

Time: 5 minutes
Serves 2

Lack of
Appetite

Nausea,
Vomiting, or
Heartburn

Constipation

Diarrhea

Fatigue

Mouth
Sores

Dry
Mouth

Chewing or
Swallowing
Difficulty

Taste
Aversion—
Sweet

Taste
Aversion—
Sour & Bitter

Lack of
Taste

Smells
Bother

Bananas and oats are good sources of soluble fiber, which helps manage diarrhea by absorbing extra fluid in the GI tract to bind the stool. They also help thicken the smoothie, making it feel almost as creamy as a milk shake.

4 Medjool dates, pitted and chopped

2 cups milk

2 medium-size frozen or fresh bananas, sliced

½ cup rolled oats

1. In a blender or food processor, puree the dates and milk until the dates are the size of small specs.
2. Add the bananas and puree until smooth.
3. Add the oats, wait for 2 to 3 minutes for the oats to soak into the mixture, then puree.
4. Pour the smoothie into two glasses and enjoy!

Nutritional Analysis: Calories 393, Total Fat 4 g, Saturated Fat 2 g, Cholesterol 12 mg, Sodium 119 mg, Carbohydrates 84 g, Dietary Fiber 8 g, Protein 13 g

Blueberry Ginger Coconut Smoothie ①

Time: 5 minutes
Serves 1

Ginger is helpful for nausea—its plant chemicals work in a similar manner as many antinausea medications to help reduce chemotherapy-induced nausea. Coconut water not only tastes delicious, but it also provides potassium and a little sugar to help you get back on track.

1 cup frozen or fresh blueberries

½ cup coconut water

1 medium-size frozen or fresh banana, sliced

1 (1-inch) piece fresh ginger, peeled and

minced, plus more to taste

Juice of 1 lime

2 tablespoons shredded unsweetened coconut

2 tablespoons walnuts

1. Place all the ingredients in a blender and blend until pureed.
2. Taste and add more ginger, if needed.
3. Pour into a glass and sip.

Nutritional Analysis: Calories 300, Total Fat 18 g, Saturated Fat 7 g, Cholesterol 0 mg, Sodium 51 mg, Carbohydrates 35 g, Dietary Fiber 8 g, Protein 4 g

Lack of Appetite	+
Nausea, Vomiting, or Heartburn	+
Constipation	+
Diarrhea	+
Fatigue	+
Mouth Sores	+
Dry Mouth	+
Chewing or Swallowing Difficulty	+
Taste Aversion—Sweet	
Taste Aversion—Sour & Bitter	+
Lack of Taste	+
Smells Bother	+

Raspberry Kiwi Julep Smoothie ◐

Time: 5 minutes
Serves 2

+	**Lack of Appetite**
+	**Nausea, Vomiting, or Heartburn**
+	**Constipation**
	Diarrhea
+	**Fatigue**
+	**Mouth Sores**
+	**Dry Mouth**
+	**Chewing or Swallowing Difficulty**
+	**Taste Aversion— Sweet**
+	**Taste Aversion— Sour & Bitter**
+	**Lack of Taste**
+	**Smells Bother**

Here's a drink that offers punch and coolness from the spearmint and lime. The rest is just water and fruit, so this is a light drink to help you stay hydrated on hot days. Plus, how can you resist the vibrant red and green colors of the raspberry and kiwi?! Omit the mint and lime if experiencing nausea or heartburn.

2 cups fresh raspberries

1 cup cold water

2 kiwis, peeled and diced

7 to 15 fresh spearmint leaves, rinsed

Juice of 1 lime

1 cup ice cubes

Honey or pure maple syrup (optional)

1. Combine the raspberries and water in a blender and puree until smooth.
2. Pour through a sieve and discard the seeds. Rinse out the blender.
3. Return the raspberry puree to the blender and add the kiwi, seven of the spearmint leaves, and the lime juice and ice cubes. Blend until smooth.
4. If desired, add honey and/or the remaining mint leaves to taste, blending after each addition.
5. Pour into two glasses and enjoy.

Nutritional Analysis: Calories 117, Total Fat 1 g, Saturated Fat 0 g, Cholesterol 0 mg, Sodium 7 mg, Carbohydrates 28 g, Dietary Fiber 11 g, Protein 3 g

Vanilla Almond Chia Seed Shake

Time: 15 minutes
Serves 2

This sweet, creamy smoothie tastes like dessert. The chia seeds are binding and create a thickness to the drink, and the vanilla and almonds add a richness that brings all the flavors together. Omit the chia seeds if experiencing gas, bloating, or lower digestive discomfort.

½ cup vanilla almond milk,
  plus more if needed

2 tablespoons chia seeds

⅓ cup toasted almonds

3 Medjool dates, pitted

3 medium-size frozen or fresh
  bananas, sliced

¼ cup plain Greek yogurt

1 teaspoon vanilla extract

1. In a small bowl, mix together the milk and chia seeds and let sit for 10 to 15 minutes.
2. Meanwhile, place the almonds and dates in a food processor or high-powered blender. Blend, scraping down the sides as you go, until the mixture becomes finely chopped and almost butterlike.
3. Add the chia seed mixture, bananas, Greek yogurt, and vanilla.
4. Blend until thick, creamy, and smooth, scraping down the sides as needed. If the shake is too thick, add more milk to your liking.
5. Pour into two glasses and enjoy.

Nutritional Analysis: Calories 463, Total Fat 17 g, Saturated Fat 2 g, Cholesterol 2 mg, Sodium 66 mg, Carbohydrates 75 g, Dietary Fiber 14 g, Protein 12 g

Lack of Appetite	+
Nausea, Vomiting, or Heartburn	+
Constipation	+
Diarrhea	
Fatigue	+
Mouth Sores	+
Dry Mouth	+
Chewing or Swallowing Difficulty	+
Taste Aversion— Sweet	
Taste Aversion— Sour & Bitter	+
Lack of Taste	+
Smells Bother	+

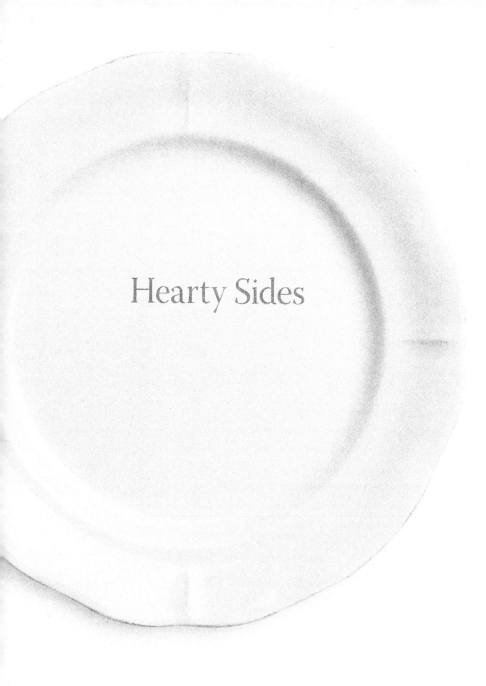

Hearty Sides

Carrot Puree with Cilantro Oil

Time: Prep: 15 minutes; Cook: 30 minutes
Serves 6 to 8

Infusing olive oil with cilantro adds just enough oomph to this simple carrot puree. Spread leftover puree over a piece of toast, for a colorful tartine. Or heat leftover puree, adding water or stock to your desired thinness, for a comforting soup.

10 medium-size carrots,
   peeled and chopped
3 tablespoons finely chopped
   fresh cilantro

5 tablespoons olive oil
Salt and freshly ground
   black pepper

1. Place carrots in a large pot and cover with water. Boil the carrots until they are very tender, for 15 to 20 minutes. Drain. Alternatively, place a steamer basket atop a pot of simmering water, add the carrots, cover, and steam for about 15 minutes, or until tender.
2. In a medium-size pan, combine the cilantro and 3 tablespoons of the olive oil. Heat over the lowest heat for about 5 minutes.
3. Remove from the heat and allow to sit for about 5 minutes. Remove and discard the cilantro, reserving the cilantro-infused oil.
4. In a food processor, combine the cooked carrots and cilantro oil and the remaining 2 tablespoons of olive oil. Puree until smooth. Add salt and pepper to taste.

Nutritional Analysis (per ½-cup serving): Calories 141, Total Fat 11 g, Saturated Fat 2 g, Cholesterol 0 mg, Sodium 150 mg, Carbohydrates 10 g, Dietary Fiber 3 g, Protein 1 g

Lack of Appetite	+
Nausea, Vomiting, or Heartburn	+
Constipation	+
Diarrhea	+
Fatigue	+
Mouth Sores	+
Dry Mouth	+
Chewing or Swallowing Difficulty	+
Taste Aversion—Sweet	+
Taste Aversion—Sour & Bitter	+
Lack of Taste	+
Smells Bother	+

Okra and Corn Succotash

Time: Prep: 15 minutes; Cook: 30 minutes
Serves 6

Lack of
Appetite

Nausea,
Vomiting, or
Heartburn

Constipation

Diarrhea

Fatigue

Mouth
Sores

Dry
Mouth

Chewing or
Swallowing
Difficulty

Taste
Aversion—
Sweet

Taste
Aversion—
Sour & Bitter

Lack of
Taste

Smells
Bother

If you have gastritis or inflammation, okra is a great food to eat. The "slime" that is typically seen with okra can coat and soothe an upset stomach. The gelatinous texture can also help those experiencing difficulty swallowing or dry mouth. If you are experiencing GI upset, omit the tomatoes as they are very acidic.

1 tablespoon olive oil

¾ cup chopped okra

4 cups fresh or frozen corn kernels

3 scallions, chopped

2 small tomatoes, chopped

2 garlic cloves, chopped

Salt and freshly ground
　　black pepper

1. Heat the olive oil in a sauté pan over medium-high heat. Add the chopped okra to the pan and cook for 3 to 5 minutes, or until it begins to soften. Add the corn to the pan, stir, and raise the theat to medium-high. Cook for about 3 minutes, until the corn begins to brown.
2. Add the scallions, tomatoes, and garlic to the pan. Stir, then cook for about 2 minutes more. Season with salt and pepper to taste and enjoy.

Nutritional Analysis (per ½-cup serving): Calories 95, Total Fat 2 g, Saturated Fat 0 g, Cholesterol 0 mg, Sodium 60 mg, Carbohydrates 20 g, Dietary Fiber 3 g, Protein 3 g

Zucchini Leek Latkes

Time: Prep: 15 minutes; Cook: 30 minutes
Makes about 6 (3-inch) latkes

Latkes are traditionally made with potatoes, but this version uses shredded zucchini and sliced leeks. Think of it like a savory pancake or fritter that is less carbohydrate dense yet has the benefit of extra nutrients. Latkes can be wrapped and frozen for up to a month, so make extra today to save time and energy another day.

¼ cup thinly sliced leeks

2 tablespoons minced garlic

3 teaspoons olive oil, or as needed

1 medium-size zucchini, grated

¼ cup all-purpose flour

1 teaspoon sugar

½ teaspoon salt

1 large egg, beaten

1 teaspoon freshly squeezed lemon juice

½ teaspoon lemon zest

1. In a medium-size skillet, sauté the leeks and garlic in 1 teaspoon of the olive oil over medium-high heat until translucent, for about 3 minutes. Remove from the heat and let cool.
2. Combine the grated zucchini, leek mixture, flour, sugar, and salt in a medium-size bowl and toss to combine. Add the egg and lemon juice and zest and stir to combine.
3. Line a plate with a layer of paper towels.
4. Heat the remaining 2 teaspoons of olive oil in a large skillet over medium-high heat.
5. Scoop the batter with a tablespoon and place in the skillet, flattening each scoop to make a 3-inch-diameter latke. Do not crowd; you will need to work in batches. Cook for about 1 minute on each side, or until the latkes have browned on both sides and are semifirm.
6. Transfer to the paper towel–lined plate and repeat until all the batter is used, adding more oil to the pan if necessary.

Nutritional Analysis (per latke): Calories 65, Total Fat 3 g, Saturated Fat 1 g, Cholesterol 36 mg, Sodium 175 mg, Carbohydrates 7 g, Dietary Fiber 1 g, Protein 2 g

Lack of Appetite	+
Nausea, Vomiting, or Heartburn	+
Constipation	+
Diarrhea	+
Fatigue	+
Mouth Sores	+
Dry Mouth	+
Chewing or Swallowing Difficulty	+
Taste Aversion—Sweet	+
Taste Aversion—Sour & Bitter	+
Lack of Taste	+
Smells Bother	+

Asian Stir-Fry with Bok Choy and Mushrooms

Time: Prep: 15 minutes; Cook: 30 minutes
Serves 2

Lack of Appetite

Nausea, Vomiting, or Heartburn

Constipation

Diarrhea

Fatigue

Mouth Sores

Dry Mouth

Chewing or Swallowing Difficulty

Taste Aversion— Sweet

Taste Aversion— Sour & Bitter

Lack of Taste

Smells Bother

Shiitake mushrooms are a source of vitamin D, which can be helpful as an extra source in the low-sun winter months. Omit the red pepper flakes and sesame oil to tone down the spice and flavor for enhanced tolerance. Mix leftover stir-fry into soba or ramen noodles, for a more substantial meal. Or make the leftovers into stock for a hearty soup.

1 tablespoon sesame or vegetable oil

1 tablespoon minced fresh ginger

3 cups baby bok choy, ends trimmed, cut into 1-inch pieces

6 fresh shiitake mushrooms, sliced into ½-inch pieces

¼ teaspoon red pepper flakes (optional)

Salt

1 teaspoon brown rice vinegar

2 tablespoons vegetable stock or water

1. Heat the sesame oil in a large skillet over medium heat.
2. Add the ginger and stir for about 15 seconds, or until fragrant. Add the bok choy, shiitake mushrooms, and red pepper flakes, if using. Sauté for a few minutes.
3. Taste and season with salt as needed.
4. Add the rice wine vinegar and sauté for about 1 minute. Add the vegetable stock and cover; cook for 3 to 4 minutes, until just tender.

Nutritional Analysis: Calories 97, Total Fat 8 g, Saturated Fat 1 g, Cholesterol 0 mg, Sodium 194 mg, Carbohydrates 7 g, Dietary Fiber 3 g, Protein 3 g

Glazed Brussels Sprouts Sauté ⓘ

Time: Prep: 10 minutes; Cook: 15 minutes
Serves 2

Glazed Brussels sprouts are a great fall side dish. Serve them atop a baked sweet potato for an eye-catching green and orange color contrast. Avoid Brussels sprouts if experiencing gas or bloating and use the glaze on 2 cups of your favorite chopped winter squash, such as acorn squash.

10 medium-size to large Brussels sprouts	1 to 2 tablespoons balsamic vinegar
1 tablespoon olive oil, plus more if needed	1 teaspoon low-sodium soy sauce
	1 tablespoon honey

1. Soak the Brussels sprouts in a bowl of cold water for 5 minutes. Drain thoroughly. Trim the ends of the Brussels sprouts and remove the outer leaves. Cut each sprout into halves or quarters, depending on their size.
2. Heat the olive oil in a skillet over medium-high heat. Add the Brussels sprouts and sauté for 2 to 3 minutes.
3. Add 2 tablespoons of water. Cover, lower the heat to low, and simmer for 3 to 5 minutes, or until the sprouts begin to soften.
4. Whisk together the balsamic vinegar, soy sauce, and honey and add to the sprouts. Cook for 3 more minutes. Serve warm.

Nutritional Analysis: Calories 157, Total Fat 7 g, Saturated Fat 1 g, Cholesterol 0 mg, Sodium 124 mg, Carbohydrates 19 g, Dietary Fiber 4 g, Protein 3 g

Symptom	
Lack of Appetite	+
Nausea, Vomiting, or Heartburn	
Constipation	+
Diarrhea	
Fatigue	+
Mouth Sores	+
Dry Mouth	+
Chewing or Swallowing Difficulty	+
Taste Aversion—Sweet	+
Taste Aversion—Sour & Bitter	+
Lack of Taste	+
Smells Bother	+

Cauliflower and Edamame "Rice"

Time: Prep: 15 minutes; Cook: 30 minutes
Serves 6

Lack of
Appetite

Nausea,
Vomiting, or
Heartburn

Constipation

Diarrhea

Fatigue

Mouth
Sores

Dry
Mouth

Chewing or
Swallowing
Difficulty

Taste
Aversion—
Sweet

Taste
Aversion—
Sour & Bitter

Lack of
Taste

Smells
Bother

A great replacement for those looking to avoid conventional rice so as to manage carbohydrate intake. For extra protein, use Bragg Liquid Aminos instead of soy sauce. Add 3 ounces of orange juice or the juice of one orange to increase the flavor.

1 medium-size head cauliflower

1½ teaspoons sesame oil

½ medium-size yellow onion,
   finely diced

½ cup fresh or frozen shelled
   edamame

4 scallions, sliced

3 tablespoons low-sodium soy sauce

1. Remove the florets from the head of cauliflower, cutting off any tough stems.
2. Transfer the florets to a food processor and pulse until the pieces have become the size of rice grains. Alternatively, grate the florets with a cheese grater—it should yield about 4 cups of cauliflower "rice." Set aside.
3. Place 1 teaspoon of the sesame oil in a large, nonstick skillet over medium heat. When the oil is hot, add the onion and cook for 4 to 5 minutes, or until the onion is soft.
4. Add the edamame and cauliflower and cook, stirring constantly, for 5 to 6 minutes, until the cauliflower is heated through.
5. Mix in the scallions, soy sauce, and remaining ½ teaspoon of sesame oil, stir until well combined, then taste for seasoning.
6. Remove from the heat and transfer to a serving dish.

Nutritional Analysis: Calories 64, Total Fat 2 g, Saturated Fat 0 g, Cholesterol 0 mg, Sodium 305 mg, Carbohydrates 9 g, Dietary Fiber 3 g, Protein 4 g

Stretch and Save: Make lettuce cups by filling large lettuce leaves with leftover cauliflower edamame rice. For added flavor, dip into a peanut sauce or Coconut Curry Sauce (page 224).

Nutritionist's Favorite to Savor
This recipe is my favorite because it has all the comfort and taste of a starchy rice dish without the added heaviness. Fiber-rich cauliflower is nicely balanced with plant-based protein from the edamame.

Hint of Cardamom Spinach Gratin

Time: Prep: 15 minutes; Cook: 30 minutes
Serves 8 to 10

For a great twist on an old favorite, this recipe adds the exotic flavor of cardamom. It is also a great high-calorie recipe for those looking to increase calories. Serve as a side dish at a holiday meal.

+	Lack of Appetite
	Nausea, Vomiting, or Heartburn
+	Constipation
	Diarrhea
+	Fatigue
+	Mouth Sores
+	Dry Mouth
+	Chewing or Swallowing Difficulty
+	Taste Aversion— Sweet
+	Taste Aversion— Sour & Bitter
+	Lack of Taste
+	Smells Bother

3 tablespoons unsalted butter
1 medium-size onion, finely chopped
¼ cup all-purpose flour
¼ teaspoon ground cardamom
3 cups milk

3 (16-ounce) packages frozen chopped spinach, defrosted and drained
¾ cup grated Pecorino Romano cheese
½ cup shredded Gruyère cheese
Salt and freshly ground black pepper

1. Preheat the oven to 425°F.
2. In a sauté pan, melt the butter over medium heat. Add the onion and sauté until translucent, for 10 to 12 minutes.
3. Add the flour and cardamom and cook for 2 more minutes, stirring occasionally. All the flour should be absorbed by the butter.
4. Add 1 cup of the milk, stirring constantly, until the flour mixture is incorporated. Add the remaining 2 cups of milk and cook, stirring constantly, until thickened slightly, for 5 to 7 minutes.
5. Squeeze as much liquid as possible from the spinach and add the spinach to the sauce.
6. Add ½ cup of the Pecorino Romano cheese and ¼ cup of the Gruyère cheese and mix well. Season with salt and pepper to taste.
7. Transfer the spinach mixture to a large baking dish, sprinkle the remaining ¼ cup of Pecorino Romano cheese and ¼ cup of the Gruyere cheese on top, and bake for 20 minutes, until hot and bubbly. Serve hot.

Nutritional Analysis (per ½-cup serving): Calories 78, Total Fat 4 g, Saturated Fat 2 g, Cholesterol 11 mg, Sodium 138 mg, Carbohydrates 6 g, Dietary Fiber 2 g, Protein 6 g

Stretch and Save: Make mini crostini with leftover gratin. Slice a baguette into thin rounds, brush with olive oil, and toast in the oven until warmed. Dollop a spoon of gratin atop the crostini bites.

Baked Eggplant Fries with Marinara Dipping Sauce

Time: Prep: 15 minutes; Cook: 30 minutes
Serves 4

How can you resist anything coated in panko bread crumbs? These eggplant fries are baked in a hot oven, not fried, making for healthy finger food at its best. Serve with marinara sauce for a classic flavor combo that's also fun to eat.

1 medium-size eggplant	1 large egg, beaten
1 teaspoon olive oil	1 cup panko bread crumbs
½ teaspoon salt	¼ cup grated Parmesan cheese
½ teaspoon freshly ground black pepper	1 cup Mirepoix Marinara Sauce (page 217), for dipping

1. Preheat the oven to 450°F. Line a baking sheet with parchment paper.
2. Cut the ends off the eggplant. Starting at one end, slice the eggplant into ¼-inch-thick slices. Cut each slice into ¼-inch strips. Be sure to cut all the strips the same size so they will cook evenly.
3. Place the eggplant strips in a bowl and season with the olive oil, salt, and pepper.
4. Place the beaten egg in a shallow bowl. Combine the panko and grated Parmesan cheese in another shallow bowl.
5. Dip a few strips of eggplant at a time into the egg, then into the panko mixture. Using a fork or your hands, remove the eggplant from the crumbs and place on the prepared baking sheet.
6. Bake for 15 to 20 minutes, or until the panko turns golden. Serve hot with warm marinara sauce for dipping. Alternatively, pour the marinara sauce over the eggplant fries and bake for another 5 minutes, until the sauce is warmed through.

Nutritional Analysis (not including marinara): Calories 154, Total Fat 4 g, Saturated Fat 1 g, Cholesterol 58 mg, Sodium 367 mg, Carbohydrates 24 g, Dietary Fiber 4 g, Protein 7 g

Nutritionist's Favorite to Savor
This recipe is my favorite because it takes an often underutilized vegetable, the eggplant, and makes it shine with a healthy coating of bread crumbs and a roast in the oven. Keeping the skin on helps reap the most nutritional benefits from the eggplant.

Symptom	
Lack of Appetite	+
Nausea, Vomiting, or Heartburn	
Constipation	+
Diarrhea	
Fatigue	+
Mouth Sores	+
Dry Mouth	+
Chewing or Swallowing Difficulty	+
Taste Aversion— Sweet	+
Taste Aversion— Sour & Bitter	+
Lack of Taste	+
Smells Bother	+

Sautéed Asparagus and Peas ①

Time: Prep: 5 minutes; Cook: 30 minutes
Serves 4 to 6

This is an easy dish to help meet the recommended minimum of five servings per day of vegetables. Add leftover asparagus and peas to a creamy risotto. The green and white colors feel so seasonal for spring!

....

2 tablespoons canola oil   asparagus, trimmed and chopped
1 shallot, minced   1 (10-ounce) bag frozen peas, thawed
1 bunch (about 1 pound) fresh   1½ tablespoons honey

....

1. Heat the canola oil in a saucepan over medium-high heat. Add the shallot and sauté for 1 to 2 minutes, until soft.
2. Add the asparagus to the pan and cook, stirring frequently to keep from burning, until cooked through and slightly golden brown on the outside.
3. Add the peas and sauté for just a few minutes until cooked.
4. Stir in the honey until well mixed.

Nutritional Analysis (per ½-cup serving): Calories 93, Total Fat 4 g, Saturated Fat 0 g, Cholesterol 0 mg, Sodium 28 mg, Carbohydrates 12 g, Dietary Fiber 3 g, Protein 3 g

+	Lack of Appetite
	Nausea, Vomiting, or Heartburn
+	Constipation
	Diarrhea
+	Fatigue
+	Mouth Sores
+	Dry Mouth
+	Chewing or Swallowing Difficulty
+	Taste Aversion— Sweet
+	Taste Aversion— Sour & Bitter
+	Lack of Taste
+	Smells Bother

Versatile Ratatouille

Time: Prep: 15 minutes; Cook: 30 minutes
Serves 4

Ratatouille makes a lovely pasta, omelet filling, or sauce for chicken or fish. Add fire-roasted tomatoes for a smokier flavor. The soft texture of this recipe is also very easy to chew and swallow for those experiencing difficulty.

1 medium-size eggplant, ends trimmed	2 medium-size bell peppers (any color), seeded and cut into large dice
1 tablespoon olive oil	
1 medium-size onion, cut into large dice	5 garlic cloves
	¼ teaspoon herbes de Provence
1 (28-ounce) can whole peeled tomatoes	¼ teaspoon salt
3 medium-size zucchini, cut into large dice	½ teaspoon freshly ground black pepper

1. Going lengthwise along the eggplant, cut into ½-inch strips, then chop it into 1-inch pieces.
2. Heat the olive oil in a large sauté pan over medium heat and sauté the onion until translucent. Add the eggplant and sauté until it becomes golden.
3. Meanwhile, in a large bowl, hand crush the whole peeled tomatoes, keeping all the juices.
4. Add the zucchini, bell peppers, and tomatoes plus their juices to the pan.
5. Stir in the whole garlic cloves, herbs, salt, and black pepper.
6. Cover with a lid and let stew for about 15 minutes. At this point, the vegetables will have reduced a bit in volume from cooking.
7. Lower the heat to medium-low and simmer for about 30 minutes. Taste and adjust the seasonings as needed.
8. Uncover, lower the heat to low, and let simmer for 20 to 30 minutes more, until most of the cooking liquid has evaporated. Taste and adjust the salt and black pepper as needed. Serve warm.

Nutritional Analysis: Calories 138, Total Fat 5 g, Saturated Fat 1 g, Cholesterol 0 mg, Sodium 558 mg, Carbohydrates 27 g, Dietary Fiber 8 g, Protein 5 g

Symptom	
Lack of Appetite	+
Nausea, Vomiting, or Heartburn	
Constipation	+
Diarrhea	
Fatigue	+
Mouth Sores	
Dry Mouth	+
Chewing or Swallowing Difficulty	+
Taste Aversion—Sweet	+
Taste Aversion—Sour & Bitter	+
Lack of Taste	+
Smells Bother	

Roasted Roots with Nutmeg Gremolata

Time: Prep: 20 minutes; Cook: 45 minutes
Serves 8

This recipe is great if you suffer from constipation; just remove the Brussels sprouts if gas and bloating are an issue, as they can be gas-producing. Toss toasted bread cubes and mozzarella cubes with leftover root veggies and gremolata to make a wintery panzanella salad.

1 pound medium-size carrots, peeled and halved crosswise, then lengthwise	4 tablespoons olive oil
	Salt and freshly ground black pepper
	¾ cup pecans
1 pound medium-size parsnips, peeled and halved crosswise, then lengthwise	1 teaspoon ground nutmeg
	¼ cup (about 1 ounce) grated Parmesan cheese
1 pound turnips, peeled, halved, cut into 1-inch-thick wedges	¼ cup finely chopped fresh parsley
1 pound Brussels sprouts, trimmed and halved	2 tablespoons freshly squeezed lemon juice
2 fennel bulbs, trimmed and cut into 1-inch thick pieces	1 tablespoon finely grated lemon zest
	1 small garlic clove, minced

1. Preheat the oven to 425°F.
2. Toss the carrots, parsnips, turnips, Brussels sprouts, and fennel in a large bowl with 3 tablespoons of the olive oil.
3. Transfer to rimmed baking sheet; sprinkle with salt and pepper.
4. Roast until the vegetables are tender, tossing often, for 40 minutes to 1 hour. Transfer the vegetables to a large platter.
5. Make the gremolata: Using a food processor, chop the pecans until coarsely ground. Transfer the ground pecans to a small bowl. Stir in the nutmeg, grated cheese, parsley, 1 tablespoon of the lemon juice, and the lemon zest, garlic, and remaining tablespoon of oil. Season to taste with salt.
6. Drizzle the vegetables with the remaining tablespoon of lemon juice.
7. Sprinkle the gremolata over the vegetables just before serving. Serve warm or at room temperature.

Lack of Appetite

Nausea, Vomiting, or Heartburn

Constipation

Diarrhea

Fatigue

Mouth Sores

Dry Mouth

Chewing or Swallowing Difficulty

Taste Aversion— Sweet

Taste Aversion— Sour & Bitter

Lack of Taste

Smells Bother

Nutritional Analysis: Calories 270, Total Fat 16 g, Saturated Fat 2 g, Cholesterol 30 mg, Sodium 170 mg, Carbohydrates 9 g, Dietary Fiber 10 g, Protein 6 g

Sautéed Vegetable Medley

Time: Prep: 15 minutes; Cook: 30 minutes
Serves 2 to 4

Lack of
Appetite

Nausea,
Vomiting, or
Heartburn

Constipation

Diarrhea

Fatigue

Mouth
Sores

Dry
Mouth

Chewing or
Swallowing
Difficulty

Taste
Aversion—
Sweet

Taste
Aversion—
Sour & Bitter

Lack of
Taste

Smells
Bother

Add your favorite seasonings—garlic, Italian seasoning, parsley, and so on—for more flavor. This vegetable medley pairs well when added to almost any dish. Mix it with eggs for a quiche, add it to pasta, or serve alongside a piece of fish.

1 tablespoon olive oil
1 yellow summer squash, sliced in half lengthwise and cut into ¼-inch half-moons
1 cup sliced mushrooms

1 cup snow peas, trimmed and cut in half
1 medium-size red bell pepper, seeded and sliced

1. Pour the olive oil into a pan over medium heat.
2. Add the squash, mushrooms, snow peas, and bell pepper and cook, stirring occasionally, until tender. Top with any of the sauces in our sauces section, such as the Kale or Basic Pesto (pages 218 and 219), Cashew Cream (page 222), or Coconut Curry Sauce (page 224).

Nutritional Analysis (per ½-cup serving): Calories 56, Total Fat 3 g, Saturated Fat 0 g, Cholesterol 0 mg, Sodium 6 mg, Carbohydrates 5 g, Dietary Fiber 2 g, Protein 2 g

Rosemary Vegetables en Papillote

Time: Prep: 15 minutes; Cook: 30 minutes
Serves 2

Add your favorite vegetables for variation. Soft, tender zucchini or summer squash would work well for diarrhea. Enjoy leftovers with a quick-cooking grain, such as quinoa or couscous. Or pile leftovers onto a roll and grill the sandwich on a skillet like a panini.

8 ounces button or cremini mushrooms, sliced	finely chopped
	1 teaspoon chopped fresh oregano
8 ounces firm tofu, diced into bite-size cubes	1½ tablespoons balsamic vinegar
	1 tablespoon olive oil
1 garlic clove, minced	Salt and freshly ground pepper
Leaves from 1 sprig of rosemary,	2 sprigs of fresh thyme (optional)

1. Preheat the oven to 400°F.
2. Cut two sheets of parchment paper, each the size of a baking sheet. Take one sheet of parchment, fold it in half, and trim edges into the shape of half a heart, so that when you unfold the paper, the paper is heart-shaped. Repeat with the other piece.
3. Combine the sliced mushrooms, tofu, garlic, rosemary, oregano, balsamic vinegar, olive oil, salt, and pepper in a large bowl and toss until the mushrooms and tofu are evenly coated.
4. Place one heart-shaped paper on one side of a baking sheet.
5. Place half of the mushroom mixture onto one side of the paper, toward the crease, trying to keep it as compact as possible. Place a thyme sprig on top, if using. Fold the other half of the heart over the mushroom mixture.
6. Starting at the top of the curve of the heart, fold the bottom edge of the paper ¼ inch over the top, pinching it off to close it. Work your way down the edge, doing the same fold, until you've sealed up the whole packet with a single fold all around. Fold the edge of the paper toward you tightly, starting at the top curve of the heart. After the first fold, take the next inch or so and fold it toward you again, overlapping the previous fold a little bit. Continue this process until you've sealed up the whole pocket with what is now a double fold all around.

Symptom	
Lack of Appetite	+
Nausea, Vomiting, or Heartburn	
Constipation	+
Diarrhea	
Fatigue	+
Mouth Sores	+
Dry Mouth	+
Chewing or Swallowing Difficulty	+
Taste Aversion— Sweet	+
Taste Aversion— Sour & Bitter	+
Lack of Taste	+
Smells Bother	+

7. Repeat the sealing process with the remaining heart and the mushroom mixture. Place the packets on a single baking sheet and bake for 20 minutes. The packets should be quite puffed up. Snip them open carefully with scissors, watching out for escaping steam, and serve.

Nutritional Analysis: Calories 209, Total Fat 13 g, Saturated Fat 2 g, Cholesterol 0 mg, Sodium 14 mg, Carbohydrates 10 g, Dietary Fiber 2 g, Protein 14 g

Sweet Potato Home Fries

Time: Prep: 15 minutes; Cook: 30 minutes
Serves 4

Home fries make a great side dish or snack anytime. Sweet potatoes pack more nutrients, such as vitamins A and C, into each bite than regular potatoes, which can help boost the immune system. Reheat leftovers and serve with eggs or salsa, or toss with colorful vegetables.

4 to 5 pounds sweet potatoes (3 or 4 large potatoes), peeled and cut into 1-inch pieces
⅓ cup olive oil

2 tablespoons minced garlic
1 cup chopped fresh parsley leaves
Salt and freshly ground black pepper

1. Preheat the oven to 450°F.
2. Bring a large pot of water to a boil and add a good pinch of salt; add the potatoes and boil until barely tender, for about 5 minutes. Meanwhile, prepare an ice bath for the potatoes.
3. Drain the potatoes, then plunge them into the ice bath to stop the cooking. When they're cool, drain again. Toss them in a large roasting pan with the olive oil and garlic.
4. Roast the potatoes, tossing them occasionally, until completely tender and lightly browned, for 15 to 20 minutes. Toss with the parsley, salt, and pepper, and serve.

Nutritional Analysis: Calories 269, Total Fat 18 g, Saturated Fat 3 g, Cholesterol 0 mg, Sodium 312 mg, Carbohydrates 25 g, Dietary Fiber 4 g, Protein 3 g

Symptom	
Lack of Appetite	+
Nausea, Vomiting, or Heartburn	+
Constipation	+
Diarrhea	+
Fatigue	+
Mouth Sores	+
Dry Mouth	+
Chewing or Swallowing Difficulty	+
Taste Aversion— Sweet	
Taste Aversion— Sour & Bitter	+
Lack of Taste	+
Smells Bother	+

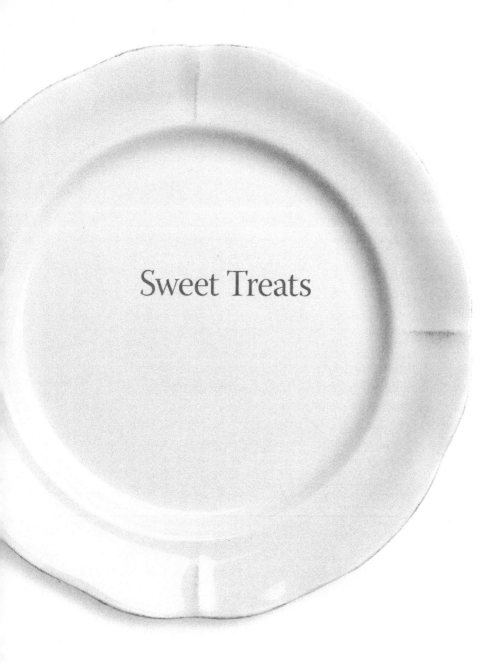

Sweet Treats

Peanut Butter Chocolate Banana Whip ◐

Time: 10 minutes
Serves 4

This recipe whips up quickly for an energy-dense treat. Leftovers (in the rare occasion that there are any) can be stored in an airtight container in the freezer for up to 2 weeks. Scoop it like ice cream! Omit or reduce chopped peanuts or chocolate chips as needed for oral or digestive sensitivity.

....

4 medium-size bananas, thinly sliced and frozen overnight

2 tablespoons peanut butter

½ cup chopped unsalted peanuts

½ cup dark chocolate chips

....

1. Combine the frozen bananas and peanut butter in a food processor. Alternatively, use a blender and stir frequently, scraping down the sides. The mixture will first look like the consistency of oats, but keep blending and soon the mixture will look like ice cream!
2. Stir in the chopped peanuts and chocolate chips.

Nutritional Analysis: Calories 399, Total Fat 22 g, Saturated Fat 8 g, Cholesterol 0 mg, Sodium 50 mg, Carbohydrates 51 g, Dietary Fiber 7 g, Protein 9 g

Lack of Appetite	+
Nausea, Vomiting, or Heartburn	+
Constipation	+
Diarrhea	+
Fatigue	+
Mouth Sores	+
Dry Mouth	+
Chewing or Swallowing Difficulty	+
Taste Aversion— Sweet	
Taste Aversion— Sour & Bitter	+
Lack of Taste	+
Smells Bother	+

Fudgy Date and Almond Truffles ◐

Time: 30 minutes
Makes 24 balls

Lack of
Appetite

Nausea,
Vomiting, or
Heartburn

Constipation

Diarrhea

Fatigue

Mouth
Sores

Dry
Mouth

Chewing or
Swallowing
Difficulty

Taste
Aversion—
Sweet

Taste
Aversion—
Sour & Bitter

Lack of
Taste

Smells
Bother

These little truffles of joy are energy packed and the fiber from the dates will help to alleviate constipation. A subtle sprinkling of powdered sugar at the end makes for a decorative touch. Leftovers can be stored in the refrigerator for up to a week or in the freezer for up to a month.

1 cup whole roasted unsalted almonds

15 Medjool dates, pitted

⅔ cup unsweetened cocoa powder

1 tablespoon honey, pure maple syrup, or agave nectar

Powdered sugar (optional)

1. In a food processor, pulse the almonds until ground.
2. Add the dates, cocoa powder, honey, and 2 tablespoons of water. Mix until it forms a sticky mass. If it seems too dry, add 1 teaspoon of water at a time. Wash your hands and lightly dry them. Using damp hands (keep the faucet running) measure out 1 tablespoon of the mixture and roll it into a ball. Set the balls on a sheet of parchment paper. Repeat until all the mixture is molded.
3. Sprinkle each with a little powdered sugar, if using.

Nutritional Analysis (per truffle): Calories 77, Total Fat 3 g, Saturated Fat 0 g, Cholesterol 0 mg, Sodium 4 mg, Carbohydrates 13 g, Dietary Fiber 2 g, Protein 2 g

Cinnamon Honey Baked Bananas

Time: Prep: 5 minutes; Cook: 15 minutes
Serves 2

These banana boats are so tasty and comforting, it almost feels like roasting fireside. For a twist, replace the honey with chocolate chips. The bananas soften as they bake, making them great for someone with chewing or swallowing difficulty.

2 medium-size ripe bananas in the peel	½ teaspoon ground cinnamon
2 teaspoons honey	¼ cup plain Greek yogurt or whipped cream

1. Preheat the oven to 400°F.
2. Wash the outside of the banana peels. For each banana, cut a lengthwise slit through the peel and halfway into the banana, but do not cut all the way through.
3. Drizzle the honey and sprinkle the cinnamon into the slit.
4. Wrap each banana in foil. Place on a baking sheet. Bake for 10 to 15 minutes, until the bananas have warmed through and softened slightly.
5. Unwrap the foil, and eat the bananas right out of the peel. Don't forget to top each banana with a dollop of Greek yogurt or whipped cream!

Nutritional Analysis (without Greek yogurt or whipped cream topping):
Calories 128, Total Fat 0 g, Saturated Fat 0 g, Cholesterol 0 mg, Sodium 1 mg, Carbohydrates 33 g, Dietary Fiber 3 g, Protein 1 g

Lack of Appetite +

Nausea, Vomiting, or Heartburn +

Constipation +

Diarrhea +

Fatigue +

Mouth Sores +

Dry Mouth +

Chewing or Swallowing Difficulty +

Taste Aversion— Sweet

Taste Aversion— Sour & Bitter +

Lack of Taste +

Smells Bother +

Frozen Banana Strawberry Bowls ①

Time: 10 minutes
Serves 4

This cool and creamy treat soothes as it goes down. Substitute a dollop of whipped cream for the walnuts if experiencing mouth sores. Or add both for a yummy dessert! Leftovers will keep in the freezer for 1 week.

4 medium-size bananas, sliced and frozen overnight	2 cups (1 pint) fresh strawberries, hulled and sliced
	Chopped walnuts

1. In a blender, combine the frozen bananas and strawberries. Blend until the mixture reaches a creamy, ice cream–like consistency, scraping down the sides as needed. Freeze or serve immediately, topped with chopped walnuts.

Nutritional Analysis (without walnuts): Calories 132, Total Fat 1 g, Saturated Fat 0 g, Cholesterol 0 mg, Sodium 2 mg, Carbohydrates 33 g, Dietary Fiber 5 g, Protein 2 g

+ Lack of Appetite

+ Nausea, Vomiting, or Heartburn

+ Constipation

+ Diarrhea

+ Fatigue

+ Mouth Sores

+ Dry Mouth

+ Chewing or Swallowing Difficulty

Taste Aversion—Sweet

+ Taste Aversion—Sour & Bitter

+ Lack of Taste

+ Smells Bother

Molten Dark Chocolate Cake

Time: Prep: 15 minutes; Cook: 30 minutes
Serves 3

Warm, ooey-gooey chocolate desserts always look impressive; just don't tell your guests how easy this one is to make. Unbaked filled ramekins can be frozen (well wrapped), and baked individually straight from the freezer whenever you like. But hold off on this recipe if you are experiencing nausea, heartburn, or gastritis, as chocolate is an irritant.

Unsalted butter and unsweetened cocoa powder, for ramekins

3 ounces 70% dark chocolate, broken into large pieces

1½ tablespoons pure maple syrup or agave nectar

1½ tablespoons unsweetened cocoa powder

½ tablespoon vanilla extract

3 tablespoons boiling water

4 tablespoons (½ stick) unsalted butter, chopped, or ¼ cup coconut oil

1 large egg

2 large egg yolks

1. Preheat the oven to 425°F. Grease the sides of three individual-size ramekins with unsalted butter and dust them with unsweetened cocoa powder.
2. In a food processor, pulse the chocolate pieces until they are crumbly.
3. Add the maple syrup, cocoa powder, and vanilla. Pulse together until the mixture has a grainy, sandlike texture.
4. Add the boiling water to the mixture, then process it again until thick and melted.
5. Add the chopped butter, egg, and egg yolks and blend until smooth and creamy.
6. Divide the batter evenly among the ramekins, then place the ramekins in the middle of the oven and bake for 10 minutes for a molten center or for 15 minutes for a completely cooked center. Let cool for 10 minutes. Invert each cake onto a plate or eat directly from the ramekins.

Nutritional Analysis: Calories 401, Total Fat 32 g, Saturated Fat 18 g, Cholesterol 256 mg, Sodium 33 mg, Carbohydrates 23 g, Dietary Fiber 4 g, Protein 7 g

Lack of Appetite	+
Nausea, Vomiting, or Heartburn	
Constipation	+
Diarrhea	+
Fatigue	+
Mouth Sores	+
Dry Mouth	+
Chewing or Swallowing Difficulty	+
Taste Aversion—Sweet	
Taste Aversion—Sour & Bitter	+
Lack of Taste	+
Smells Bother	+

Mini Ricotta Coconut Fruit Pies with Hazelnut Crust

Time: Prep: 15 minutes; Cook: 30 minutes
Makes 6 small or 12 mini tarts

Lack of
Appetite

+ Nausea,
Vomiting, or
Heartburn

+ Constipation

Diarrhea

+ Fatigue

Mouth
Sores

+ Dry
Mouth

+ Chewing or
Swallowing
Difficulty

Taste
Aversion—
Sweet

+ Taste
Aversion—
Sour & Bitter

+ Lack of
Taste

+ Smells
Bother

This is an impressive tart that doesn't even require turning on the oven! The crust is naturally sweetened with dates and is made from pulsed oats and hazelnuts, held together with coconut oil and omega-3-rich flaxseeds. The filling is a delicious creamy mix of ricotta cheese and coconut milk. Top with your favorite chopped fruits.

For the crust

½ cup rolled or quick oats

½ cup hazelnuts

¼ teaspoon salt

15 Medjool dates, pitted and chopped (¾ cup chopped)

¼ cup coconut oil, or 4 tablespoons unsalted butter

1 teaspoon vanilla extract

1 tablespoon ground flax or chia seeds

For the filling and toppings

¼ cup + 2 tablespoons canned coconut milk

½ cup (4 ounces) part-skim ricotta cheese

½ tablespoon honey

Fruit toppings of choice, such as raspberries, strawberries, kiwi, and mango, thinly sliced (keep raspberries whole or cut in half)

1. Grind the oats in a food processor or blender to make an oat flour. Transfer to a large bowl.
2. Place the hazelnuts and salt in the food processor and grind until the nuts start to resemble a coarse flour. Add to the oats.
3. Place the dates in the food processor and pulse until very finely chopped. Add the oat flour mixture back and pulse together with the dates (you may need to do this in batches, depending on the size of your food processor or blender).
4. Add the coconut oil and vanilla. Pulse a few times, pushing the mixture down with a spoon between pulses.
5. When the mixture is mostly smooth and sticky like dough, transfer to a bowl and mix in the ground flaxseeds. You should be able to touch the dough without it getting stuck all over your hands, although your hands may be greasy after working with it.

6. Press the dough into twelve mini muffin cups, six standard muffin cups, or six individual tart molds. Alternatively, press the dough into a 9-inch pie or tart pan. Place the muffin tins or tart pan(s) in the freezer for at least 1 to 2 hours to help the crusts hold their shape.
7. In a saucepan over low to medium heat, gently heat the coconut milk for about 2 minutes, stirring constantly so that it does not burn. Set aside to cool to room temperature.
8. Beat the ricotta cheese, coconut milk, and honey with an electric mixer until smooth.
9. Remove the crusts from the molds and fill with a few spoons of the filling and top with sliced fruit. Store the finished fruit pies in the fridge.

Nutritional Analysis (for 1 small tart or 2 mini tarts; does not include fruit topping): Calories 343, Total Fat 18 g, Saturated Fat 12 g, Cholesterol 6 mg, Sodium 118 mg, Carbohydrates 47 g, Dietary Fiber 5 g, Protein 6 g

Secret Ingredient Chocolate Banana Pudding ⓘ

Time: 15 minutes
Serves 2

+	Lack of Appetite
+	Nausea, Vomiting, or Heartburn
+	Constipation
+	Diarrhea
+	Fatigue
+	Mouth Sores
+	Dry Mouth
+	Chewing or Swallowing Difficulty
	Taste Aversion— Sweet
+	Taste Aversion— Sour & Bitter
+	Lack of Taste
+	Smells Bother

Tofu is the secret ingredient in this pudding, giving this dessert a smooth, silky texture and a good dose of protein. Freezing the pudding into Popsicles makes for a soothing treat for a dry mouth. Don't have a Popsicle mold? Use an ice cube tray with Popsicle sticks to make mini Popsicles. Leftovers can be covered and stored in the freezer for 1 day. Reblending or stirring the ingredients the next day may help re-create a smooth consistency. Those sensitive to chocolate can reduce or omit as needed.

2 medium-size frozen or fresh bananas, sliced

5 ounces silken tofu

¼ cup regular or soy milk (use chocolate milk for added sweetness)

2 tablespoons agave nectar, honey, or sugar

2 tablespoons unsweetened cocoa powder

1 teaspoon vanilla extract

1. Combine all the ingredients in a blender and puree until smooth.
2. Pour into two glasses and enjoy.

Nutritional Analysis: Calories 237, Total Fat 3 g, Saturated Fat 1 g, Cholesterol 0 mg, Sodium 20 mg, Carbohydrates 49 g, Dietary Fiber 5 g, Protein 7 g

Dark Chocolate–Coated PB & B Truffles ⓘ

Time: 30 minutes
Makes 20 truffles

Talk about a functional food, these decadent truffles made with peanut butter, banana, and cereal are a great way to help meet daily fiber intake and to alleviate constipation. Best enjoyed within 3 to 5 days.

1 cup fiber cereal	1 tablespoon agave nectar or honey
¾ cup creamy peanut butter	(optional)
1 medium-size banana,	6 ounces dark chocolate, broken
sliced	into pieces

1. In a food processor, grind the cereal into fine crumbs.
2. Add the peanut butter, banana, and agave nectar, if using, and pulse for a few times until the dough comes together.
3. Roll the dough into small balls and place them on a parchment paper–lined cookie sheet. Transfer to the refrigerator for about an hour.
4. Melt the chocolate in a double boiler (a glass bowl on top of a saucepan with simmering water works). Once melted, move the bowl of chocolate to a work surface and submerge each truffle in the chocolate. Use a spoon to scoop out each truffle and let excess chocolate drip off before placing on the parchment paper.
5. Place in the refrigerator, unwrapped, to allow the chocolate to set. Once set, store in a covered container in the refrigerator.

Nutritional Analysis: Calories 122, Total Fat 9 g, Saturated Fat 3 g, Cholesterol 0 mg, Sodium 55 mg, Carbohydrates 9 g, Dietary Fiber 2 g, Protein 3 g

Lack of Appetite +

Nausea, Vomiting, or Heartburn

Constipation +

Diarrhea

Fatigue +

Mouth Sores +

Dry Mouth +

Chewing or Swallowing Difficulty +

Taste Aversion— Sweet

Taste Aversion— Sour & Bitter +

Lack of Taste +

Smells Bother +

Chocolate Avocado Fudgsicles

Time: 15 minutes prep; 5 hours freeze
Serves 4

Lack of
Appetite

Nausea,
Vomiting, or
Heartburn

Constipation

Diarrhea

Fatigue

Mouth
Sores

Dry
Mouth

Chewing or
Swallowing
Difficulty

Taste
Aversion—
Sweet

Taste
Aversion—
Sour & Bitter

Lack of
Taste

Smells
Bother

Avocados and nuts add healthy fats to a classic Fudgsicle. If you do not have Popsicle molds, use an ice cube tray with Popsicle sticks to make mini Fudgsicles. Note that the avocado flavor is slightly more pronounced when the pops are frozen. To tone down the avocado notes, simply enjoy the mixture as a pudding and store it in the refrigerator. Avoid the nuts and pretzels if you have difficulty chewing or swallowing or mouth sores. Leftover Fudgsicles will last in the freezer for up to 5 days. Those sensitive to chocolate can reduce or omit as needed.

2 large ripe avocados, peeled
  and pitted
⅔ cup unsweetened cocoa powder
½ cup honey or agave nectar
¼ teaspoon vanilla extract

Suggested topping: chopped
  pistachios, walnuts, or peanuts;
  shredded coconut; or crushed
  chocolate-covered pretzels

1. Place the avocados, cocoa powder, honey, vanilla extract, and ¼ cup of water in a blender. Blend until light and fluffy, adding a little more water if a little stiff.
2. Enjoy chilled as a pudding, or divide among four Popsicle molds and let set in the freezer for at least 5 hours, or until frozen.
3. Enjoy once frozen or roll the slightly softened Popsicles in nuts, coconut, pretzels, or all three!

Nutritional Analysis (does not include toppings): Calories 321, Total Fat 17 g, Saturated Fat 3 g, Cholesterol 0 mg, Sodium 11 mg, Carbohydrates 51 g, Dietary Fiber 11 g, Protein 5 g

Chocolate Raspberry Pudding ◑

Time: 15 minutes
Serves 4

Not straining the raspberry seeds adds fiber and texture. To prevent a skin from forming on the top of pudding, place a layer of plastic wrap directly on top of the pudding before storing in in the refrigerator. Those sensitive to chocolate can reduce or omit as needed.

....

2 cups milk

1 cup fresh or frozen raspberries

2 tablespoons unsweetened cocoa
   powder

3 tablespoons cornstarch

1 teaspoon sugar

¼ teaspoon vanilla extract

1 tablespoon pure maple syrup

Fresh berries, to serve

Toasted almonds, chopped, to serve

....

1. Place all the ingredients (except the fresh berries and almonds) in a blender and blend until smooth.
2. Pour this mixture into a small saucepan and heat over medium heat, stirring frequently, until it bubbles and thickens. This will take several minutes.
3. As soon as the pudding has thickened, remove the saucepan from the heat and place it in an ice bath. The ice water should reach about halfway up the saucepan. Stir frequently to help the pudding cool and prevent a skin from forming.
4. Scoop the chilled pudding into four serving bowls or glasses and top with the berries and almonds.

Nutritional Analysis (not including toppings): Calories 114, Total Fat 2 g, Saturated Fat 1 g, Cholesterol 6 mg, Sodium 56 mg, Carbohydrates 21 g, Dietary Fiber 3 g, Protein 5 g

Stretch and Save: Make icebox cakes with leftover pudding. Place a layer of graham crackers or wafer cookies in a pan, adding a layer of pudding on top, another layer of cookies, and another layer of pudding. Store in the refrigerator overnight; the next day, the cookies will have softened into cakelike layers. Yum!

Lack of Appetite	+
Nausea, Vomiting, or Heartburn	+
Constipation	+
Diarrhea	
Fatigue	+
Mouth Sores	+
Dry Mouth	+
Chewing or Swallowing Difficulty	+
Taste Aversion— Sweet	
Taste Aversion— Sour & Bitter	+
Lack of Taste	+
Smells Bother	+

Creamy Coconut Popsicles

Time: Prep: 5 minutes; Freeze time: 2 hours minimum
Makes 10 Popsicles

+	Lack of Appetite
+	Nausea, Vomiting, or Heartburn
+	Constipation
+	Diarrhea
+	Fatigue
+	Mouth Sores
+	Dry Mouth
+	Chewing or Swallowing Difficulty
	Taste Aversion— Sweet
+	Taste Aversion— Sour & Bitter
+	Lack of Taste
+	Smells Bother

Sweet coconut is a delicious treat in any form, but especially as a cool, soothing Popsicle. Cardamom adds a unique twist but may need to be reduced or omitted if you are experiencing nausea. Leftover Popsicles will last in the freezer for up to 5 days.

½ cup powdered sugar

1 (14-ounce) can light coconut milk

1 (12-ounce) can fat-free evaporated milk

⅛ teaspoon ground cardamom

½ cup shredded sweetened coconut

1. In a bowl, mix the powdered sugar with half of the coconut milk until it is incorporated.
2. Add the other half of the coconut milk and the rest of the ingredients and whisk together. Pour into ten Popsicle molds. Freeze overnight and enjoy.

Nutritional Analysis: Calories 103, Total Fat 4 g, Saturated Fat 4 g, Cholesterol 2 mg, Sodium 63 mg, Carbohydrates 13 g, Dietary Fiber 0 g, Protein 3 g

Dark Chocolate Raisin Oat Flour Cookies ◑

Prep time: 15 minutes; Cook time: 15 minutes
Makes 18 to 20 cookies

A great treat to make ahead and use as an on-the-go snack. To make your own oat flour, use a food processor, blender, or coffee grinder: blend enough rolled oats to equal 3 cups of ground flour. Don't want to bake all the cookies now? Roll extra dough into a log and freeze. Slice off the ends of the log, as desired, as they can go directly from the freezer into the oven for baking. Those sensitive to chocolate can reduce or omit as needed.

8 tablespoons (1 stick) unsalted butter, at room temperature	½ tablespoon vanilla extract
½ cup packed light brown sugar	2 large eggs
½ cup granulated sugar	3 cups oat flour
1 teaspoon baking soda	½ cup raisins
½ teaspoon salt	½ cup dark chocolate chunks or chips

1. Preheat the oven to 375°F and line two baking sheets with parchment paper.
2. In a large bowl, cream the butter and sugars. Continue to mix until well combined and creamy, with no visible chunks of butter.
3. Mix in the baking soda, salt, vanilla, and eggs, scraping down the side of the bowl as needed. Add the oat flour and continue to mix until the dough comes together. Once the ingredients are combined, stir in the raisins and chocolate until eventually distributed.
4. Scoop the dough into balls, roughly the size of 2 heaping tablespoons, and set on the prepared baking sheet. Press the balls down slightly.
5. Bake for 12 to 14 minutes, or until the cookies are golden on top. Remove from the oven and let cool on the baking sheet.

Nutritional Analysis: Calories 183, Total Fat 8 g, Saturated Fat 4 g, Cholesterol 35 mg, Sodium 129 mg, Carbohydrates 26 g, Dietary Fiber 2 g, Protein 3 g

♥ Nutritionist's Favorite to Savor
This recipe is my favorite because it takes a basic chocolate chip cookie and replaces refined all-purpose flour with oat flour, boosting the soluble fiber in the recipe for easier digestion and health. Yes, you can still have your cookie and eat it, too!

Symptom	
Lack of Appetite	+
Nausea, Vomiting, or Heartburn	+
Constipation	+
Diarrhea	+
Fatigue	+
Mouth Sores	
Dry Mouth	
Chewing or Swallowing Difficulty	+
Taste Aversion—Sweet	
Taste Aversion—Sour & Bitter	+
Lack of Taste	+
Smells Bother	+

Whipped Sweet Potato Pie ①

Time: Prep: 10 minutes; Cook time: 15 minutes
Serves 4

Here's a lightened-up crustless sweet potato pie, thanks to a filling made with coconut milk. Sprinkle with crushed graham crackers or gingersnap cookies, and add a dollop of whipped cream if you're feeling indulgent. Extra mashed sweet potatoes can be used in the Sweet Potato and Broccoli Mac and Cheese (page 105).

2 sweet potatoes, peeled and chopped, or 1 cup mashed cooked sweet potato
½ cup full-fat coconut milk
1 tablespoon sugar, honey, or pure maple syrup, or more to taste

¼ teaspoon ground cinnamon
¼ teaspoon ground nutmeg
¼ teaspoon ground ginger
Crushed graham crackers or gingersnap cookies, for serving

1. If using fresh sweet potatoes, boil until tender, for 8 to 12 minutes. Drain the water, let cool slightly, and mash potatoes with a hand mixer until smooth. Scoop out 1 cup of the mash and place in a bowl for use in the recipe (enjoy any leftovers separately).
2. Warm the coconut milk and slowly add to the sweet potato mash, stirring as you go. To get the mixture extra smooth, use an immersion blender to whip the mixture.
3. Mix in the sugar and spices until well combined.
4. Pour the mixture into four individual cups.
5. Top with crushed graham crackers. Enjoy immediately.

Nutritional Analysis (not including crushed graham crackers or ginger snaps): Calories 134, Total Fat 6 g, Saturated Fat 5 g, Cholesterol 0 mg, Sodium 52 mg, Carbohydrates 19 g, Dietary Fiber 1 g, Protein 2 g

Nutritionist's Favorite to Savor
This recipe is my favorite because it is a dessert that can be enjoyed by all at the holiday table. Using coconut milk instead of cream gives this whipped crustless pie a rich flavor that can be tolerated by those who are experiencing dairy intolerance. Plus, I always enjoy an opportunity to eat vegetables for dessert.

Sidebar (left margin):

- Lack of Appetite
- Nausea, Vomiting, or Heartburn
- Constipation
- Diarrhea
- Fatigue
- Mouth Sores
- Dry Mouth
- Chewing or Swallowing Difficulty
- Taste Aversion—Sweet
- Taste Aversion—Sour & Bitter
- Lack of Taste
- Smells Bother

Ginger Granita

Time: Prep: 30 minutes + an overnight freeze
Serves 8 (makes 4 cups granita)

A light and refreshing treat for a hot summer day. Or, if feeling nauseated, as ginger is helpful in reducing chemotherapy-induced nausea. Granita will keep in the freezer for up to 5 days.

3 tablespoons peeled and thickly sliced fresh ginger
1½ cups sugar

2 teaspoons freshly squeezed lemon juice

1. Chill a baking pan for 2 hours in the freezer.
2. In a blender or food processor, puree the ginger with 1 cup of water.
3. Combine the ginger puree, sugar, and 2½ cups of water in a saucepan. Bring to a bare simmer over high heat, stirring frequently, not allowing the mixture to boil.
4. Strain the mixture through a fine-mesh strainer, reserving the liquid and discarding the pulp.
5. Stir in the lemon juice and pour into the prechilled baking pan. Place on a level surface in the freezer.
6. Let the mixture freeze overnight until solid.
7. Use a metal spoon to scrape the mixture into a light, granular texture or place broken pieces in a food processor and chop to your desired texture.

Nutritional Analysis (per ½-cup serving): Calories 116, Total Fat 0 g, Saturated Fat 0 g, Cholesterol 0 mg, Sodium 4 mg, Carbohydrates 30 g, Dietary Fiber 0 g, Protein 0 g

Lack of Appetite	+
Nausea, Vomiting, or Heartburn	+
Constipation	+
Diarrhea	+
Fatigue	+
Mouth Sores	
Dry Mouth	+
Chewing or Swallowing Difficulty	+
Taste Aversion— Sweet	+
Taste Aversion— Sour & Bitter	+
Lack of Taste	+
Smells Bother	+

Juicy Grilled Summer Peaches ◑

Time: Prep: 5 minutes; Cook: 10 minutes
Serves 4

Serve this light and healthy treat with yogurt or ice cream for an energy-dense snack or dessert. Place leftover peaches between two graham crackers with a small dollop of yogurt, or add a piece of chocolate and eat it like a s'more! This recipe also works great with nectarines, plums, pears, or apples.

....

4 peaches, halved and pitted
1 tablespoon honey or agave
 nectar
1 teaspoon vanilla extract

2 tablespoons freshly squeezed
 lemon juice
½ teaspoon ground cinnamon
Zest of 1 lemon

....

1. Heat grill to medium-low heat.
2. Place the peach halves, cut side up, on a large sheet of heavy-duty foil.
3. In a small bowl, mix together the honey, vanilla, lemon juice, and cinnamon. Spread the mixture evenly upon all the peach halves.
4. Fold the foil tightly over the peaches, ensuring that there is a tight seal.
5. Grill for 15 to 18 minutes, or until the peaches are tender. Alternatively, roast the peaches in a preheated 400°F oven for 15 minutes, until tender. More time may be needed, depending on how tender the peaches were to begin with.
6. Carefully open the foil pouches and allow the steam to escape.
7. Garnish with lemon zest and serve immediately.

Nutritional Analysis: Calories 80, Total Fat 0 g, Saturated Fat 0 g, Cholesterol 0 mg, Sodium 0 mg, Carbohydrates 19 g, Dietary Fiber 2 g, Protein 1 g

---

+	Lack of Appetite
+	Nausea, Vomiting, or Heartburn
+	Constipation
+	Diarrhea
+	Fatigue
+	Mouth Sores
+	Dry Mouth
+	Chewing or Swallowing Difficulty
+	Taste Aversion— Sweet
	Taste Aversion— Sour & Bitter
+	Lack of Taste
+	Smells Bother

Staple Sauces & Condiments

Tomato Habanero Salsa ①

Time: 15 minutes
Serves 6

This salsa is great if you like spicy food! When handling a hot pepper, such as a habanero, be sure to wear gloves or wash your hands well after touching the pepper. The spice can get on your skin and can cause a very painful stinging sensation if you touch an eye or your face. Serve this salsa with tortilla chips or inside your favorite taco, burrito, quesadilla, or tostada.

3 medium-size tomatoes, chopped

¼ cup chopped scallions

1 small red onion, finely chopped

½ cup chopped fresh cilantro

1 habanero pepper, finely chopped

2 garlic cloves, minced

Juice of 1 lime

½ teaspoon salt

1. Place all the ingredients in a large bowl and stir to mix.
2. Chill for about 30 minutes to let the flavors develop.

Nutritional Analysis: Calories 19, Total Fat 0 g, Saturated Fat 0 g, Cholesterol 0 mg, Sodium 164 mg, Carbohydrates 4 g, Dietary Fiber 1 g, Protein 1 g

Lack of
Appetite

Nausea,
Vomiting, or
Heartburn

Constipation

Diarrhea

Fatigue

Mouth
Sores

Dry
Mouth

Chewing or
Swallowing
Difficulty

Taste
Aversion—
Sweet

Taste
Aversion—
Sour & Bitter

Lack of
Taste

Smells
Bother

Pineapple Mango Salsa ⓘ

Time: 15 minutes
Serves 6

Grilling the pineapple gives it a charred, sweeter taste. This salsa is sweet and savory all in one. The bright yellow and orange colors from the pineapple and mango look dashing next to the red and green colors of the herbs and vegetables. Serve with Cinnamon Pear Chips (page 165), for a unique tasty treat!

2 teaspoons olive oil

½ ripe pineapple, peeled, cored, and sliced into 1-inch-thick slices

1 mango, peeled, pitted, and diced

¼ medium-size red onion, minced

2 scallions, thinly sliced

3 tablespoons chopped fresh cilantro

3 tablespoons freshly squeezed lime juice

1 tablespoon honey

A few dashes of hot sauce (optional)

Salt and freshly ground black pepper

1. Heat the olive oil in a grill pan or large skillet over medium-high heat. Grill the pineapple for about 2 minutes per side, or until lightly charred. Remove from the heat and set aside to cool.
2. Finely chop the cooled pineapple slices and place in a small bowl.
3. In a large bowl, stir together the diced mango, onion, scallions, cilantro, lime juice, and honey. Add the chopped pineapple. Season with a few dashes of hot sauce, if using, and salt and pepper to taste.
4. Chill in the refrigerator for at least 30 minutes to let the flavors develop.

Nutritional Analysis: Calories 101, Total Fat 2 g, Saturated Fat 0 g, Cholesterol 0 mg, Sodium 83 mg, Carbohydrates 23 g, Dietary Fiber 2 g, Protein 1 g

Lack of Appetite	+
Nausea, Vomiting, or Heartburn	
Constipation	+
Diarrhea	
Fatigue	+
Mouth Sores	
Dry Mouth	+
Chewing or Swallowing Difficulty	+
Taste Aversion—Sweet	
Taste Aversion—Sour & Bitter	
Lack of Taste	+
Smells Bother	+

Yogurt Hollandaise Sauce ①

Time: 15 minutes
Makes 1 cup sauce

Hollandaise gets a lighter makeover by using yogurt instead of butter. Make your own fancy brunch at home by topping this Yogurt Hollandaise atop the Red and Green Eggs Florentine (page 49). Or drizzle the sauce over roasted asparagus, for a classic seasonal spring dish.

1 cup plain yogurt
2 teaspoons freshly squeezed lemon
   juice
3 large egg yolks

½ teaspoon salt
½ teaspoon Dijon mustard
Freshly ground black pepper
Fresh dill, for garnish

1. In a medium-size bowl, beat the yogurt, lemon juice, and egg yolks well.
2. In a double boiler or a glass bowl placed on top of a saucepan of simmering water, heat the yogurt mixture, stirring frequently, until the sauce has thickened slightly, for about 20 minutes.
3. Remove from the heat and stir in the salt, mustard, and pepper to taste. The sauce will continue to thicken as it cools. Top with fresh dill.

Nutritional Analysis (per 2-tablespoon serving): Calories 40, Total Fat 2 g, Saturated Fat 1 g, Cholesterol 71 mg, Sodium 152 mg, Carbohydrates 3 g, Dietary Fiber 0 g, Protein 3 g

Nutritionist's Favorite to Savor
This recipe is my favorite because it is a unique way to add calories and protein to dishes for those who need an extra bite. This recipe uses calcium-rich yogurt in place of the traditional butter that is often called for in hollandaise recipes.

Sidebar symptoms list:
- \+ Lack of Appetite
- \+ Nausea, Vomiting, or Heartburn
- \+ Constipation
- \+ Diarrhea
- \+ Fatigue
- \+ Mouth Sores
- \+ Dry Mouth
- \+ Chewing or Swallowing Difficulty
- \+ Taste Aversion— Sweet
- \+ Taste Aversion— Sour & Bitter
- \+ Lack of Taste
- \+ Smells Bother

Cucumber Tzatziki ①

Time: 15 minutes
Makes 1 cup sauce

Savory yogurt, also known as tzatziki, is a signature staple of many Mediterranean dishes. Try it in the Greek Grilled Salmon with Tzatziki (page 140), or serve it as a dip with your favorite crudité vegetables. Omit the vinegar if you have mouth sores or sensitivity. Yogurt can otherwise have a very cooling effect on the mouth.

1 medium-size cucumber, washed, unpeeled, and seeded
1 cup plain Greek yogurt
1 garlic clove, finely minced
1 tablespoon freshly squeezed lemon juice
1 teaspoon salt
½ tablespoon red wine vinegar
1 tablespoon olive oil
Freshly ground black pepper
1 tablespoon chopped fresh dill, mint, or parsley (optional)

1. Grate the cucumber, retaining as much of the juice as you can.
2. In a medium-size bowl, add the cucumber and its juices to the yogurt.
3. Whisk in the garlic, lemon juice, salt, red wine vinegar, and olive oil. Add pepper to taste and the herbs, if using.
4. Let the tzatziki chill in the refrigerator for at least 30 minutes to let the flavors develop.

Nutritional Analysis (per ¼-cup serving): Calories 52, Total Fat 3 g, Saturated Fat 1 g, Cholesterol 3 mg, Sodium 334 mg, Carbohydrates 3 g, Dietary Fiber 0 g, Protein 3 g

Lack of Appetite	+
Nausea, Vomiting, or Heartburn	+
Constipation	+
Diarrhea	+
Fatigue	+
Mouth Sores	+
Dry Mouth	+
Chewing or Swallowing Difficulty	+
Taste Aversion— Sweet	+
Taste Aversion— Sour & Bitter	
Lack of Taste	+
Smells Bother	+

Aromatic Vegetable Stock

Time: Prep: 15 minutes; Cook: 1–1½ hours
Makes 2 quarts stock

Lack of
Appetite

Nausea,
Vomiting, or
Heartburn

Constipation

Diarrhea

Fatigue

Mouth
Sores

Dry
Mouth

Chewing or
Swallowing
Difficulty

Taste
Aversion—
Sweet

Taste
Aversion—
Sour & Bitter

Lack of
Taste

Smells
Bother

Making your own vegetable stock is so much tastier and better for you than buying it from the store. Add whatever vegetable odds and ends you have lying around. Make it your own by tossing in your favorite herbs and spices, too. The stock can be made 3 days ahead. Let cool completely, then cover and chill, or freeze for up to 3 months. Freeze the stock in ice cube trays for quicker thawing. Once frozen, transfer the stock ice cubes to a bag. Six ice cubes equals about ½ cup thawed stock.

1 tablespoon olive oil
2 medium-size onions, unpeeled,
　　cut into 1-inch pieces
10 celery ribs, cut into 1-inch pieces
2 large carrots, peeled, cut into
　　1-inch pieces
8 ounces cremini or button mushrooms,
　　halved

1 small fennel bulb, cut into
　　1-inch pieces
1 head garlic, halved crosswise
6 sprigs flat-leaf parsley
1 bay leaf
1 teaspoon whole black
　　peppercorns

1. Heat the olive oil in a large stockpot over medium-high heat.
2. Add the remaining ingredients and cook, stirring occasionally, until the vegetables begin to soften, for 5 to 7 minutes.
3. Add 4 quarts of cold water. Bring to a boil, then lower the heat and simmer until the stock is reduced by half, for 1 to 1½ hours.
4. Strain the stock through a fine-mesh sieve into a large bowl; discard the solids.

Nutritional Analysis: Calories 122, Total Fat 4 g, Saturated Fat 1 g, Cholesterol 0 mg, Sodium 133 mg, Carbohydrates 20 g, Dietary Fiber 5 g, Protein 4 g

Mirepoix Marinara Sauce

Time: Prep: 15 minutes; Cook: 45 minutes
Makes 4 cups sauce

Mirepoix is a traditional French mixture of finely chopped onion, carrot, and celery. It is the base for many soups and sauces. A bunch of recipes in this cookbook call for marinara, so make this your go-to sauce! Add cooked ground turkey or chicken to make a higher-protein Bolognese sauce.

....

2 tablespoons olive oil	1 bay leaf
1 medium-size yellow onion, finely diced	¼ teaspoon dried oregano
1 medium-size carrot, finely diced	2 (28-ounce) cans crushed tomatoes
1 celery rib, finely diced	¼ teaspoon sugar
3 garlic cloves, minced	Salt and freshly ground black pepper
⅛ teaspoon red pepper flakes	⅓ cup chopped fresh basil

....

1. In a large pot, heat the olive oil over medium-high heat. Add the onions and sauté until translucent, for about 5 minutes.
2. Add the carrots and celery. Sauté until the vegetables are soft, for about 7 minutes. Add the garlic, red pepper flakes, bay leaf, and oregano and sauté for 1 minute.
3. Stir in the tomatoes and the sugar. Simmer, uncovered, for about 30 minutes, or until the vegetables are tender.
4. Remove from the heat and discard the bay leaf. Taste the sauce and season with salt and pepper, if necessary. Stir in the fresh basil.

Nutritional Analysis: Calories 155, Total Fat 4 g, Saturated Fat 1 g, Cholesterol 0 mg, Sodium 214 mg, Carbohydrates 25 g, Dietary Fiber 4 g, Protein 7 g

Lack of Appetite	+
Nausea, Vomiting, or Heartburn	
Constipation	+
Diarrhea	+
Fatigue	+
Mouth Sores	
Dry Mouth	+
Chewing or Swallowing Difficulty	+
Taste Aversion— Sweet	+
Taste Aversion— Sour & Bitter	+
Lack of Taste	+
Smells Bother	+

Kale Pesto ①

Time: 15 minutes
Serves 4

Think of this as your winter pesto. Kale lends a heartier note to pesto and is great stirred into a soup, tossed into pasta, or dolloped onto cooked vegetables or chicken.

....

1 bunch kale (about 12 ounces), stemmed and roughly chopped

2 garlic cloves, roughly chopped

¼ cup olive oil

2 tablespoons freshly squeezed lemon juice

½ cup grated Parmesan cheese

Salt and freshly ground black pepper

....

1. Place all the ingredients in a food processor, adding salt and pepper to taste. Puree until pasty and well combined, for 30 to 60 seconds.
2. Scrape into a lidded container and store in the refrigerator until ready to use.

Nutritional Analysis (per 2-tablespoon serving): Calories 284, Total Fat 22 g, Saturated Fat 7 g, Cholesterol 20 mg, Sodium 588 mg, Carbohydrates 11 g, Dietary Fiber 1 g, Protein 13 g

+ Lack of Appetite

Nausea, Vomiting, or Heartburn

+ Constipation

Diarrhea

+ Fatigue

Mouth Sores

+ Dry Mouth

+ Chewing or Swallowing Difficulty

+ Taste Aversion— Sweet

+ Taste Aversion— Sour & Bitter

+ Lack of Taste

+ Smells Bother

Basic Pesto ◖

Time: 15 minutes
Makes 1 cup pesto

Find fresh basil at its peak in the warmer summer months. Here, it gets blended with almonds instead of the more traditional pine nuts. Stir pesto into almost anything, for a fresh, punchy seasoning. Try it in the Tofu Scramble with Pesto and Roasted Cherry Tomatoes (page 60), or the Whole Wheat Couscous Primavera (page 114).

½ cup whole almonds

½ cup olive oil

½ tablespoon freshly squeezed
   lemon juice

2 cups basil, large stems removed

⅓ cup grated Pecorino Romano or
   Parmesan cheese

2 garlic cloves, roughly chopped

½ teaspoon salt

¼ teaspoon freshly ground
   black pepper

¼ teaspoon red pepper flakes
   (optional)

1. In a food processor or blender, process the almonds until they have turned into fine crumbs.
2. Add the remaining ingredients and process until smooth.
3. Scrape into lidded container and store in the refrigerator until ready to use.

Nutritional Analysis (per 2-tablespoon serving): Calories 139, Total Fat 14 g, Saturated Fat 2 g, Cholesterol 2 mg, Sodium 127 mg, Carbohydrates 2 g, Dietary Fiber 1 g, Protein 3 g

Symptom	
Lack of Appetite	+
Nausea, Vomiting, or Heartburn	
Constipation	+
Diarrhea	
Fatigue	+
Mouth Sores	
Dry Mouth	+
Chewing or Swallowing Difficulty	+
Taste Aversion— Sweet	+
Taste Aversion— Sour & Bitter	+
Lack of Taste	+
Smells Bother	+

Dijon Balsamic Dressing ◑

Time: 15 minutes
Makes 1 cup dressing

This is an easy dressing to whisk up and pour over any salad. Or try something different to wake up the taste buds—use this as a dip for French fries instead of ketchup.

....

1 tablespoon Dijon mustard
4 tablespoons olive oil
4 tablespoons balsamic vinegar
1 garlic clove, minced

1 tablespoon freshly squeezed
   lemon juice
1 tablespoon chopped fresh basil
Salt and freshly ground black pepper

....

Whisk together all the ingredients in a bowl, adding salt and pepper to taste. Pour on top of your favorite salad, veggies, or pasta.

Nutritional Analysis: Calories 34, Total Fat 4 g, Saturated Fat 1 g, Cholesterol 0 mg, Sodium 32 mg, Carbohydrates 1 g, Dietary Fiber 0 g, Protein 0 g

+ Lack of
  Appetite

Nausea,
Vomiting, or
Heartburn

+ Constipation

Diarrhea

+ Fatigue

Mouth
Sores

+ Dry
  Mouth

+ Chewing or
  Swallowing
  Difficulty

Taste
Aversion—
Sweet

+ Taste
  Aversion—
  Sour & Bitter

+ Lack of
  Taste

+ Smells
  Bother

Mediterranean Artichoke Olive Sauce

Time: Prep: 15 minutes; Cook: 30 minutes
Serves 4

Artichokes are such an underrated vegetable. Not only do they provide a unique flavor, but they are also extremely nutritious. This sauce goes well with the Your Way Zucchini Noodles (page 104) or any whole-grain pasta you prefer.

1 cup artichoke hearts, halved	1 tablespoon white wine
½ cup pitted kalamata olives, halved	vinegar
3 tablespoons olive oil	3 garlic cloves, minced
Zest of 1 lemon	2 tablespoons chopped fresh
3 tablespoons freshly squeezed	parsley
lemon juice	½ teaspoon salt, or to taste

Whisk together all the ingredients in a small bowl.

Nutritional Analysis: Calories 200, Total Fat 18 g, Saturated Fat 2 g, Cholesterol 0 mg, Sodium 804 mg, Carbohydrates 9 g, Dietary Fiber 3 g, Protein 1 g

Stretch and Save: Make quick Mediterranean flatbreads with leftover sauce. Lay slices of pita on a baking sheet and brush with the sauce and some feta cheese. Bake in a preheated 375°F oven or the toaster oven until heated through.

Symptom	
Lack of Appetite	+
Nausea, Vomiting, or Heartburn	
Constipation	+
Diarrhea	
Fatigue	+
Mouth Sores	
Dry Mouth	+
Chewing or Swallowing Difficulty	+
Taste Aversion— Sweet	+
Taste Aversion— Sour & Bitter	
Lack of Taste	+
Smells Bother	

Cashew Cream ◔

Time: 15 minutes
Makes 2 cups cashew cream

This recipe is a gem! Adds smooth, creamy protein to many recipes. Savory cashew cream makes a great pasta sauce or dipping sauce, and it tastes great with Carrot Ginger Soup (page 155). Sweet cashew cream can be turned into a parfait by layering the cream with nuts, fruit, and jam in a jar.

2 cups raw cashews

1 cup cold water, plus more
   as needed

½ to ¾ teaspoon salt (optional)

1 to 2 tablespoons freshly squeezed
   lemon juice

2 tablespoons pure maple syrup
   (optional)

1. Soak the cashews in cold water for at least 6 hours or overnight.
2. Drain cashews. Add them to a food processor with the cup of cold water and blend, stopping a few times to scrape down the bowl. Depending on how thick or thin you want the cream, keep adding water until you like the consistency.
3. For a savory cream, add the salt and lemon juice. For a sweet cream, add the maple syrup. Feel free to vary the flavorings as you like!

Nutritional Analysis (per 2-tablespoon serving): Calories 79, Total Fat 6 g, Saturated Fat 1 g, Cholesterol 0 mg, Sodium 3 mg, Carbohydrates 4 g, Dietary Fiber 0 g, Protein 2 g

---

Lack of Appetite +

Nausea, Vomiting, or Heartburn

Constipation +

Diarrhea

Fatigue +

Mouth Sores +

Dry Mouth +

Chewing or Swallowing Difficulty +

Taste Aversion—Sweet

Taste Aversion—Sour & Bitter

Lack of Taste +

Smells Bother +

Supersmooth Ginger Hummus

Time: 15 minutes
Makes 2 cups hummus

Adding lemon zest and grated fresh ginger gives this hummus a real zing. Use hummus as a snack or small meal if trying to consume small, frequent meals to manage symptoms. Reduce the lemon if experiencing mouth soreness.

1 (15-ounce) can chickpeas, drained and rinsed

2 tablespoons tahini

2 tablespoons olive oil, plus more for serving

2 garlic cloves, finely chopped

1 teaspoon grated fresh ginger

Zest of 1 lemon

Juice of ¼ lemon

Salt

1. Reserving a few chickpeas for garnish, place all the ingredients plus 2 tablespoons of water in a blender, adding salt to taste.
2. Blend and add more water, as needed, to get the hummus to your desired thickness. When serving, toss the reserved chickpeas on top and drizzle with a little olive oil.

Nutritional Analysis: Calories 125, Total Fat 6 g, Saturated Fat 1 g, Cholesterol 0 mg, Sodium 220 mg, Carbohydrates 15 g, Dietary Fiber 3 g, Protein 4 g

Nutritionist's Favorite to Savor
This recipe is my favorite because it takes a popular dip, hummus, and gives it a special lemon ginger flavor that is especially compatible with those who suffer from lack of taste and nausea. Forgo the store-bought hummus and make your own.

Symptom	
Lack of Appetite	+
Nausea, Vomiting, or Heartburn	+
Constipation	+
Diarrhea	+
Fatigue	+
Mouth Sores	+
Dry Mouth	+
Chewing or Swallowing Difficulty	+
Taste Aversion— Sweet	+
Taste Aversion— Sour & Bitter	+
Lack of Taste	+
Smells Bother	+

Coconut Curry Sauce

Time: Prep: 15 minutes; Cook: 30 minutes
Serves 4

The curry powder in this sauce will make the whole house smell cozy and warm. Serve this sauce over sautéed vegetables and grains, or use it as a marinade for tofu, shrimp, or chicken.

Lack of
Appetite

Nausea,
Vomiting, or
Heartburn

Constipation

Diarrhea

Fatigue

Mouth
Sores

Dry
Mouth

Chewing or
Swallowing
Difficulty

Taste
Aversion—
Sweet

Taste
Aversion—
Sour & Bitter

Lack of
Taste

Smells
Bother

1¼ cups light coconut milk

2 tablespoons soy sauce

2 teaspoons sugar, or to taste

½ teaspoon salt, or to taste

2 tablespoons olive oil

1 teaspoon red pepper flakes

Zest of 1 lemon

1½ tablespoons minced garlic

1 to 1½ tablespoons curry powder

½ cup chopped fresh Thai basil leaves

1. In a small bowl, combine the coconut milk, soy sauce, sugar, and ½ teaspoon of salt.
2. Heat the olive oil in a skillet over medium-high heat. Add the red pepper flakes, lemon zest, garlic, and curry powder and stir-fry until fragrant, for about 15 seconds.
3. Add the coconut milk mixture and bring to a boil. Cook until the sauce thickens slightly, for 1½ minutes. Add the Thai basil.

Nutritional Analysis: Calories 130, Total Fat 11 g, Saturated Fat 4 g, Cholesterol 0 mg, Sodium 616 mg, Carbohydrates 9 g, Dietary Fiber 1 g, Protein 1 g

Tofu Ricotta ⓘ

Makes 2 cups ricotta

Tofu ricotta makes a great addition to a dairy-free lasagne or pizza. Or try spreading it over toast to make crostini.

1 (14-ounce) package extra-firm tofu	1 teaspoon dried oregano
2 teaspoons olive oil	2 garlic cloves
½ teaspoon salt	1 tablespoon nutritional yeast

1. Drain the tofu and pat dry with paper towels.
2. Crumble the tofu into a food processor or high-speed blender along with the olive oil, salt, oregano, garlic, and nutritional yeast. Process on high speed until smooth and ricotta-like. Alternatively, mix everything together with a fork to get a more rustic texture.

Nutritional Analysis: Calories 76, Total Fat 4 g, Saturated Fat 1 g, Cholesterol 0 mg, Sodium 224 mg, Carbohydrates 1 g, Dietary Fiber 0 g, Protein 8 g

Lack of Appetite	+
Nausea, Vomiting, or Heartburn	+
Constipation	+
Diarrhea	+
Fatigue	+
Mouth Sores	+
Dry Mouth	+
Chewing or Swallowing Difficulty	+
Taste Aversion—Sweet	+
Taste Aversion—Sour & Bitter	+
Lack of Taste	+
Smells Bother	+

Common Nutrition Topics

Nutrition has become a popular topic in today's world and, with that, it seems everyone has an opinion on what is healthy (or not). New studies are released frequently purporting to have evidence of clinical efficacy or even cure. Watch out for any diet or nutritional strategy that promises a "miracle cure" or has other "medical benefits." There is a lot of confusion about such topics as "hormone free," "antibiotic free," and "organic." There is no one-size-fits-all solution for anyone—the most important thing to keep in mind is to eat a well-balanced diet. The proper balance of calories, proteins, fats, carbohydrates, and other nutrients is the key to maintaining optimal health. Often, working with an oncology registered dietitian is a great starting point to do this safely and effectively. In this section we will help you begin to determine the healthiest foods that are right for you.

Deciphering Animal Protein Labeling

Meats, poultry, and eggs are not raised the same as they were raised in the past. Advances in technology have brought less expensive, more efficient ways of farming and raising animals, such as factory farms, battery cages, and growth hormones. These techniques are not always best for our health. Here, we break down some of the buzz words in the industry.

Grass Fed: Usually pertains to cows and means that they were fed grass rather than animal or corn feed. Grass is what cows are supposed to eat. In fact, cows are known as ruminants because the largest pouch of the stomach is called the rumen. It is essentially a 55-gallon container to help them better digest plant material giving us all of those good nutrients we love! Grass-fed beef is also a good source of conjugated linolenic acid (CLA), which is a potentially beneficial type of fatty acid.

Hormone or Antibiotic Free: While hormones were never allowed in poultry, pork, or goats, growth hormones can be given to cows and antibiotics can be given to all animals. A label stating this means that a flock or herd was raised without the use of these drugs. This is important because it is believed that the drugs used in animals could, in turn, affect our immune and endocrine systems, causing antibiotic resistance and hormonal imbalances, among other unknown effects.

Free Range: The term *free range* can be applied to poultry or eggs and is not a certification or regulated term, such as *organic*. The USDA only regulates this label term requirement for poultry to be called free range and requires that animals have access to the outdoors for some period of time per day.

Cage Free: This label indicates that the animals were not in cages and were able to freely roam a building and practice their innate behaviors; however, unlike free range they may not necessarily have access to the outdoors. This is also not a regulated USDA label term.

Natural: According to the USDA, for meat, poultry, or egg product to be labeled "natural," it must contain no artificial ingredients, coloring ingredients, or chemical preservatives and is minimally processed. This label does not account for farming practices as does the "organic" certification.

Organic: To be certified organic by the USDA, farms and ranches must follow strict guidelines, and they have to be practicing organically for a minimum of three years. Some of the other key requirements are no drugs, antibiotics, or growth hormones allowed; animals must have year-round outdoor access; animals must be fed organic feed for their entire lives; and they must be raised on certified organic pastures. Many small farms may practice organic methods but do not have the money to pay for the expensive certification.

In a perfect world everyone would be able to use organic meats, poultry, or eggs; however, these products are more expensive than their regular counterparts, often double the cost. If you are not able to buy organic, try looking at natural meats or meats without hormones and antibiotics and always try to buy lean cuts of meat, as they are lower in fat content. If you are unsure whether something at the grocery store contains added hormones and anti-biotics, feel free to ask a butcher, he or she will be happy to help.

Organic vs. Nonorganic Produce

Many cancer patients feel that organic produce is a requirement for a healthy diet and this is often a source of confusion and anxiety. Organic produce is grown without the use of pesticides and therefore helps to reduce exposure to pesticide residues and may have better nutrient retention. Since organic produce can be more expensive and harder to find for some people, it is important to remember that it is still important to consume fruits and vegetables. An excellent way to choose the safest produce and fruits and vegetables is to use the resources of the Environmental Working Group. Each year they create a list of the fifteen cleanest produce (Clean 15) items and the twelve fruits or vegetables with the highest amounts of pesticide residues (Dirty Dozen). In short, the Clean 15 are considered the safest to buy nonorganic and the Dirty Dozen includes the ones to always buy organic, if possible, to reduce your exposure to pesticide residues. This list is extremely valuable in helping the health conscious consumer select the more important organic picks to suit their budget and health needs. Visit http://www.ewg.org/foodnews/summary.php for the most up-to-date information.

Juicing vs. Blending

Juicing can be a good way to consume a variety of vegetables and fruit and help the body absorb some key vitamins and minerals. However, juices may be less filling than whole vegetables and fruits and contain less fiber because all of the juice is squeezed out of the fruit or vegetable without including the pulp or other nonfluid matter. Fruit juice in particular can contribute more calories and sugar to the diet, if large amounts are consumed. In moderation, juices can be part of a healthy diet as long as they are not a replacement for whole fruits and vegetables.

Blending is equivalent to creating a smoothie and involves putting fruit and/or vegetables in a blender and blending the entire fruit, juice, pulp, and all. It includes every part of the fruit and/or vegetable; nothing is separated out, so a smoothie contains fiber, which slows down digestion and optimizes nutrient intake. Since nothing is removed in a smoothie, these blended drinks contain more vitamins, minerals, fiber, and phytonutrients than juices because the entire fruit and/or vegetable is included. Smoothies are a great way to include more fruits and vegetables in the diet, especially for those who may have difficulty digesting whole fruits and vegetables.

Commercially juiced or blended products should be made from 100 percent vegetable or fruit juices and should be pasteurized to eliminate harmful microorganisms. Homemade juices should be used within 24 hours to ensure food safety.

Soy

Soy is a popular topic of controversy because of the contradictory research regarding its use and the development of certain types of hormone-sensitive cancers, commonly breast cancer. As such, it is an important topic for cancer patients as they think about their nutritional health. Soy contains phytochemicals called phytoestrogens. Phytoestrogens have chemical structures similar to those in human estrogen, yet there is a question as to whether or not they have similar effects in the body. In relation to breast cancer risk, research suggests that initiating soy consumption during childhood and adolescence may be beneficial. However, research of soy consumption in adulthood has revealed mixed results, likely because there are many complex factors that can affect phytoestrogen action in the body, such as metabolism, menopausal status, and age.

Women with a history of hormone-related cancers can safely consume natural whole soy foods, such as tofu, soybeans, tempeh, and soy milk, in moderation. It is recommended to limit *processed* soy foods, soy supplements, vegetarian soy-based meat alternatives, soy chips, and soy-fortified cereals. Processed soy does not contain a proper balance of nutrients and often also contains preservatives, colorings, and excessive sodium. *It is important to speak with your health-care team regarding your individual needs.*

Nutrition for Survivorship

Many patients complete cancer treatment and then wonder, "Now what"? Believe it or not, this is when the power of nutrition can have an even greater impact in helping reduce risk of recurrence. Many guidelines have been established, by organizations that include the American Institute for Cancer

Research and the American Cancer Society, to help cancer survivors make healthier diet and lifestyle choices. These guidelines recommend choosing a more plant-based diet rich in fruits, vegetables, grains, nuts, and seeds; achieving and maintaining a healthy weight; avoiding excess sodium, sugar, and processed foods; limiting red meats; increasing physical activity; limiting alcohol intake; and avoiding dietary supplements that claim to prevent cancer.

Remember that Mother Nature created plant foods as a natural way of cleansing our body and protecting it from potentially harmful carcinogens. A diet rich in colorful plant foods provides a wealth of antioxidants and phytochemicals that can neutralize oxidative damage to cells and strengthen the immune system to fight disease. Following, we highlight the benefits of some of our favorite plant foods.

Color of Fruit or Vegetable	Phytochemicals	Fruits and Vegetables
White and green	Allyl sulfides	Onions, garlic, chives, leeks
Green	Sulforaphanes, indoles	Broccoli, Brussels sprouts, cabbage, cauliflower
Yellow and green	Lutein, zeaxanthin	Asparagus, collard greens, spinach, winter squash
Orange and yellow	Cryptoxanthin, flavonoids	Cantaloupe, nectarines, oranges, papayas, peaches
Orange	Alpha- and beta-carotenes	Carrots, mangoes, pumpkin
Red and purple	Anthocyanins, polyphenols	Berries, grapes, plums
Red	Lycopene	Tomatoes, pink grapefruit, watermelon

Source: HEAL Well Guide; savorhealth.com

To make a specific cancer survivorship plan, locate the registered dietitian and cancer survivorship program coordinator at your cancer center.

Safe Food Handling

Safe food handling is an important component of healthy cooking for everyone, but *especially* for the cancer patient. This is because many cancer treatments can weaken the immune system, making it more susceptible to infection, including that from food. Many aspects of food preparation can introduce unnecessary bacteria, especially if you are unaware of the appropriate steps to follow. By following the guidelines outlined in this chapter, the introduction of potentially harmful bacteria can be avoided just by being more aware when you purchase, store, clean, prepare, thaw, cook, serve, and reheat your foods.

Purchasing Food

When shopping for food, select nonperishable foods first, and then purchase refrigerated or frozen foods at the end of the shopping trip. Never choose meat or poultry in packaging that is torn and leaking. Do not buy food past the "sell-by," or "use-by" date. Carefully check the package condition of shelf-stable foods. If the packaging has been torn or the container is dented, do not purchase. Put raw meat and poultry into a plastic bag so that juices will not contaminate other foods. Plan to drive directly home from the grocery store. You may want to pack a cooler or a bag of ice during warmer months, to keep groceries at a safe temperature.

Storage of Food

Always refrigerate perishable food within 2 hours of being cooked (1 hour when the temperature is above 90°F). Check the temperature of your refrigerator and freezer with an appliance thermometer. The refrigerator should be at 40°F or below and the freezer should be at 0°F or below. Cook or freeze fresh poultry, fish, ground meat, and variety meats within 2 days of purchase and other beef, veal, lamb, and pork within 2 to 5 days of purchase. Perishable food, such as meat and poultry, should be wrapped securely to maintain quality and prevent juices from dripping onto other foods.

To maintain quality when freezing meat and poultry in its original package, wrap the package again with foil or plastic wrap that is recommended for the freezer. High-acid canned foods, such as tomatoes, grapefruit, and pineapple, can be stored on the shelf for 12 to 28 months. Low-acid canned foods, such as meat, poultry, fish, and most vegetables, will keep for 2 to 5 years if the can remains in good condition and has been stored in a cool, clean, and dry place. Discard cans that are dented, leaking, bulging, or rusted, or that have been stored past their marked expiration date.

Cleaning Produce

Before eating or preparing, wash fresh produce under cold running tap water to remove any excess dirt. If there is a firm surface or skin on produce, such as apples, melons, or potatoes, the surface can be scrubbed with a brush. Discard the outer leaves of leafy vegetables, such as lettuce and cabbage.

The FDA has not approved the use of detergent or soap to wash fruits and vegetables. However, commercial produce washes are safe and effective. They are designed to remove soil, wax, and pesticides. A homemade rinse can be made with 1 cup of vinegar and 2 cups of cold water in a spray bottle, and used to spray produce prior to rinsing well with water.

When preparing fruits and vegetables, cut away any damaged or bruised areas because bacteria can grow in these crevices. Immediately refrigerate any fresh-cut items, such as salad or fruit, for food safety and best quality. Store produce on a shelf or in a drawer that is above raw meat so that there is no risk of meat juice dripping onto and contaminating the produce.

Preparation

Always wash your hands before and after handling food.

Do not cross-contaminate. Keep raw meat, poultry, fish, and their juices away from other foods. After cutting raw meat, wash your hands and the knife, countertop/surface, and cutting board with hot, soapy water. Use a separate cutting board for meats and for vegetables. Always sanitize cutting boards after use (in a hot dishwasher or in a solution of 1 teaspoon of chlorine bleach in 1 quart of water).

Thawing

Foods should never be thawed or stored on the counter, outdoors, or defrosted in hot water because this allows the food to reach the danger zone (40° to 140°F) in which harmful bacteria can grow. The refrigerator allows for slow thawing. Make sure thawing meat and poultry juices do not drip on other foods. For faster thawing, place the food in a leakproof plastic bag. Submerge in cold tap water. Change the water every 30 minutes. Cook immediately.

Cooking

Harmful bacteria are destroyed when food is cooked to the proper temperature. Be sure to buy a meat thermometer because this is the only reliable way to ensure safety and that the food is cooked to the proper temperature.

Proper Internal Cooking Temperature for Meats

- When roasting meat and poultry, use an oven temperature no lower than 325°F.
- Cook ground meats to 160°F; ground poultry to 165°F.
- Beef, veal, lamb steaks, roasts, and chops may be cooked to 145°F.
- All cuts of fresh pork must be 160°F.
- Whole poultry should reach 180°F in the thigh and 170°F in the breast.
- Reheat hot dogs, cold cuts, and deli-style meats to steaming before consumption, since cold luncheon meats can harbor dangerous bacteria for someone with a weakened immune system.
- Reheat leftovers to 165°F.

Serving

Hot food should be kept at 140°F or warmer. Cold food should be kept at 40°F or cooler. When serving food at a buffet, keep food hot with chafing dishes, slow cookers, and warming trays. Keep food cold with nesting dishes in bowls of ice or use small serving trays and replace them often.

Perishable food should *not* be left out for more than 2 hours at room temperature (1 hour when the temperature is above 90°F).

Leftovers

Discard any food left out at room temperature for more than 2 hours (1 hour when the temperature is above 90°F). Place the food into shallow containers and immediately put in the refrigerator or freezer for rapid cooling. Use cooked leftovers within 3 to 4 days (1 day for bone marrow transplant patients).

Refreezing

Meat and poultry defrosted in the refrigerator may be refrozen before or after cooking. If thawed by other methods cook before refreezing.

If you have any questions about how you should include food safety into your daily routine, be sure to speak with your health-care team.

Helpful References

Equivalents and Metric Conversions

The recipes in this book have not been tested with metric measurements, so some variations might occur.

Remember that the weight of dry ingredients varies according to the volume or density factor: 1 cup of flour weighs far less than 1 cup of sugar, and 1 tablespoon doesn't necessarily hold 3 teaspoons.

GENERAL FORMULA FOR METRIC CONVERSION

Ounces to grams	multiply ounces by 28.35
Grams to ounces	multiply ounces by 0.035
Pounds to grams	multiply pounds by 453.5
Pounds to kilograms	multiply pounds by 0.45
Cups to liters	multiply cups by 0.24
Fahrenheit to Celsius	subtract 32 from Fahrenheit temperature, multiply by 5, divide by 9
Celsius to Fahrenheit	multiply Celsius temperature by 9, divide by 5, add 32

OVEN TEMPERATURE EQUIVALENTS, FAHRENHEIT (F) AND CELSIUS (C)

100°F = 38°C
200°F = 95°C
250°F = 120°C
300°F = 150°C
350°F = 180°C
400°F = 205°C
450°F = 230° C

WEIGHT (MASS) MEASUREMENTS

1 ounce = 30 grams
2 ounces = 55 grams
3 ounces = 85 grams
4 ounces = ¼ pound = 125 grams
8 ounces = ½ pound = 240 grams
12 ounces = ¾ pound = 375 grams
16 ounces = 1 pound = 454 grams

LINEAR MEASUREMENTS

½ in = 1½ cm
1 inch = 2½ cm
6 inches = 15 cm
8 inches = 20 cm
10 inches = 25 cm
12 inches = 30 cm
20 inches = 50 cm

Volume (Dry) Measurements

¼ teaspoon = 1 milliliter

½ teaspoon = 2 milliliters

¾ teaspoon = 4 milliliters

1 teaspoon = 5 milliliters

1 tablespoon = 15 milliliters

¼ cup = 59 milliliters

⅓ cup = 79 milliliters

½ cup = 118 milliliters

⅔ cup = 158 milliliters

¾ cup = 177 milliliters

1 cup = 225 milliliters

4 cups or 1 quart = 1 liter

½ gallon = 2 liters

1 gallon = 4 liters

Volume (Liquid) Measurements

1 teaspoon = ⅙ fluid ounce = 5 milliliters

1 tablespoon = ½ fluid ounce = 15 milliliters

2 tablespoons = 1 fluid ounce = 30 milliliters

¼ cup = 2 fluid ounces = 60 milliliters

⅓ cup = 2 ⅔ fluid ounces = 79 milliliters

½ cup = 4 fluid ounces = 118 milliliters

1 cup or ½ pint = 8 fluid ounces = 250 milliliters

2 cups or 1 pint = 16 fluid ounces = 500 milliliters

4 cups or 1 quart = 32 fluid ounces = 1,000 milliliters

1 gallon = 4 liters

Cooking Conversions

Measures	Equivalent
Teaspoons	
Under ⅛ teaspoon	Dash or pinch
1½ teaspoons	½ tablespoon
3 teaspoons	1 tablespoon
Tablespoons	
1 tablespoon	3 teaspoons
4 tablespoons	¼ cup
5⅓ tablespoons	⅓ cup
8 tablespoons	½ cup
16 tablespoons	1 cup
Cups	
¼ cup	4 tablespoons
⅓ cup	5⅓ tablespoons
½ cup	8 tablespoons or ¼ pint
1 cup	16 tablespoons or ½ pint
2 cups	1 pint
4 cups	1 quart
Liquid Measures	
2 tablespoons	1 fluid ounce
3 tablespoons	1 jigger or 1½ fluid ounces
¼ cup	2 fluid ounces
½ cup	4 fluid ounces
1 cup	8 fluid ounces

Food to Measurement Conversion Guide

Amount	Measure
Berries or Tomatoes	
1 pint	2¼ cups
Butter or Margarine	
½ stick	¼ cup or 4 tablespoons
1 pound	4 sticks or 2 cups
Cheese	
8 ounces cream cheese	1 cup
8 ounces cottage cheese	1 cup
4 ounces Parmesan, grated	1¼ cups
Cream	
1 cup heavy cream	2 cups whipped
Dried Beans and Peas	
1 cup	2¼ cups cooked
Herbs	
1 tablespoon fresh	1 teaspoon dried
Pasta	
8 ounces macaroni	4 cups cooked
8 ounces medium-wide	3¾ cups cooked
8 ounces fine noodles	5½ cups cooked
8 ounces spaghetti	4 cups cooked
Rice	
1 cup white	3 cups cooked
1 cup converted	4 cups cooked
1 cup instant	1½ cups cooked
1 cup brown	3 to 4 cups cooked
Sugar	
1 lb granulated	2 cups
1 lb brown, firmly packed	2¼ cups
1 lb powdered sugar	4½ cups

Recipe Substitution Guide

Recipe calls for . . .	Substitute
1 square unsweetened chocolate	3 tablespoons unsweetened cocoa powder + 1 tablespoon butter
1 cup cake flour	1 cup less 2 tablespoons all-purpose flour
2 tablespoons flour (for thickening)	1 tablespoon cornstarch
1 teaspoon baking powder	¼ teaspoon baking soda + ½ teaspoon cream of tartar + ¼ teaspoon cornstarch
1 cup buttermilk	1 tablespoon of vinegar or lemon juice + enough milk to make 1 cup
1 cup sour cream	1 cup plain yogurt
1 cup firmly packed brown sugar	1 cup granulated sugar + 2 tablespoons molasses
1 teaspoon lemon juice	¼ teaspoon vinegar (not balsamic)
1 clove garlic	¼ teaspoon garlic powder
2 cups tomato sauce	¾ cup tomato paste + 1 cup water

Food Purchasing Amount Translation Guide

When the recipe calls for . . .	You need
4 cups shredded cabbage	1 small cabbage
1 cup grated raw carrot	1 large carrot
2½ cups sliced carrots	1 lb raw carrots
4 cups cooked cut fresh green beans	1 lb beans
1 cup chopped onion	1 large onion
4 cups sliced raw potatoes	4 medium-size potatoes
1 cup chopped sweet pepper	1 large pepper
1 cup chopped tomato	1 large tomato
2 cups canned tomatoes	16 ounce can
4 cups sliced apples	4 medium-size apples
1 cup mashed banana	3 medium-size bananas
1 teaspoon lemon zest	From 1 medium-size lemon
2 tablespoons lemon juice	From 1 medium-size lemon
4 teaspoons orange zest	From 1 medium-size orange
2 cups shredded Swiss or Cheddar	8 ounces cheese
1 cup egg whites	From 6 or 7 large eggs
1 cup soft bread crumbs	From 2 slices of bread

Other References

Savor Health: A technology-enabled provider of personalized nutrition resources for cancer patients and their caregivers. www.savorhealth.com. 888-721-1014.

Food safety for cancer patients: http://www.fda.gov/downloads/Food/Foodborne IllnessContaminants/UCM312761.pdf.

Oncology Nutrition Dietetic Practice Group of the Academy of Nutrition and Dietetics. M. Lesser, N. Ledesma, S. Bergerson, E. Truillo. "Oncology Nutrition for Clinical Practice." Oncology Nutrition Dietetic Practice Group of the Academy of Nutrition and Dietetics: 2013.

American Dietetic Association. *Oncology Toolkit.* Chicago, IL: American Dietetic Association: 2010. https://www.eatright.org/shop/product.aspx?id=6442472065.

World Cancer Research Fund/American Institute for Cancer Research. "Food, Nutrition, Physical Activity, and the Prevention of Cancer: A Global Perspective." Washington, DC: AICR, 2009.

L. H. Kushi, C. Doyle, M. McCullough, C. Rock, W. Denmark-Wahnefried, E. V. Bandera, S. Gapstur, A. V. Patel, K. Andrews, T. Gansler, and the American Cancer Society 2010 and Nutrition and Physical Activity Guidelines Advisory Committee. "American Cancer Society Guidelines on Nutrition and Physical Activity for Cancer Prevention: Reducing the Risk of Cancer with Healthy Food Choices and Physical Activity." *CA: A Cancer Journal for Clinicians* 62 (2012): 30–66.

C. Rock, C. Doyle, E. V. Denmark-Wahnefried, J. Meyerhardt, K. Courneya, A. Schwartz, E. Bandara, K. Hamilton, B. Grant, M. McCollough, T. Byers, and T. Gansler. "Nutrition and Physical Activity Guidelines for Cancer Survivors." *CA: A Cancer Journal for Clinicians* 62 (2012): 242–74.

HEAL Well Guide: www.savorhealth.com.

Recipes by Side Effect and Symptom

SWEET MORNINGS

	Lack of Appetite	Nausea, Vomiting, or Heartburn	Constipation	Diarrhea	Fatigue	Mouth Sores	Dry Mouth	Chewing or Swallowing Difficulty	Taste Aversion—Sweet	Taste Aversion—Sour & Bitter	Lack of Taste	Smells Bother
Apple Crumble Baked Oatmeal	+	+	+	+	+	+	+	+			+	+
Sweet Baked Banana Oatmeal	+	+	+	+	+	+	+	+		+	+	+
AB & B Oats	+	+	+	+	+	+	+	+			+	+
Simple Amaranth Porridge	+	+	+	+	+	+	+	+				+
Raw Blended Buckwheat and Chia Porridge with Raspberries, Apples, and Kiwi	+		+		+	+	+	+			+	+
Berry Banana Nut Butter Bowl	+	+	+		+		+	+			+	+
Maple Berry Breakfast Parfait	+	+	+		+		+	+		+	+	+
Peach Cardamom Honeyed Yogurt	+	+	+		+		+	+			+	+
Pineapple and Papaya "Brûlée"	+		+		+			+	+		+	+
Quinoa Coconut Pancakes	+	+	+	+	+	+			+			+
Apple Butternut Squash Yogurt Pancakes	+	+	+	+	+	+	+	+	+		+	+
Eggless Banana Battered French Toast	+	+	+	+	+	+	+	+	+	+	+	+
Cinnamon Whole Wheat Waffles	+	+	+		+	+	+			+	+	+
Multi-Bran Sour Cream Muffins	+	+	+		+	+	+		+		+	+

	Lack of Appetite	Nausea, Vomiting, or Heartburn	Constipation	Diarrhea	Fatigue	Mouth Sores	Dry Mouth	Chewing or Swallowing Difficulty	Taste Aversion—Sweet	Taste Aversion—Sour & Bitter	Lack of Taste	Smells Bother
Classic Avocado Toast	+	+	+	+	+					+	+	+
Bull's-Eye Skillet Avocado Eggs	+		+	+	+	+	+	+		+	+	+
Easy-Bake Grab-and-Go Veggie Egg Muffins	+		+		+	+	+	+	+		+	+
Red and Green Eggs Florentine	+		+		+		+	+		+	+	+
Roasted Breakfast Potatoes with Tofu Egg Scramble	+		+		+		+	+	+	+	+	+
Speedy Spinach Breakfast Tacos	+		+		+		+	+		+	+	
Eggy Quinoa Patties	+	+	+		+	+	+	+		+	+	+
Sweet or Savory Matzoh Brei	+	+	+	+	+	+	+	+		+	+	+
Cracked Eggs in Zucchini-Corn-Lime Sauté	+		+		+		+	+	+	+	+	+
Cauliflower Crust Quiche	+		+		+	+	+	+		+	+	+
Sweet Potato, Tomato, and Spinach Hash	+		+		+		+	+		+	+	
Tofu Scramble with Pesto and Roasted Cherry Tomatoes	+		+		+		+	+		+	+	
Seitan, Apple, and Broccoli Breakfast Hash	+		+		+			+		+	+	+
Vegan Mushroom Breakfast Burritos	+		+		+	+	+	+		+	+	
Chicken, Apple, and Maple Breakfast Patties	+	+	+	+	+	+	+	+		+	+	

	Lack of Appetite	Nausea, Vomiting, or Heartburn	Constipation	Diarrhea	Fatigue	Mouth Sores	Dry Mouth	Chewing or Swallowing Difficulty	Taste Aversion—Sweet	Taste Aversion—Sour & Bitter	Lack of Taste	Smells Bother
Quinoa Bowl with Sliced Avocado and Yogurt Dressing	+	+	+		+		+	+	+		+	+
Very Veggie Farro Salad	+		+		+		+		+		+	
Warm Lima Bean and Aspara-gus Salad with Arugula Parsley Pesto	+		+		+		+				+	
Thai Style Vegeta-ble Strand Salad	+		+		+		+		+		+	+
Carrot, Date, and Chickpea Salad	+		+		+		+			+	+	
Drunken Feta Caprese Salad	+		+		+		+	+	+		+	
Summery Black Bean, Jicama, and Corn Salad	+		+		+		+				+	
Red Cabbage Slaw with Pecans and Double Citrus Dressing	+		+		+		+			+	+	
Creamy Avocado Egg Salad	+		+	+	+	+	+	+			+	
Chicken Salad with Celery and Grapes	+	+	+		+		+			+	+	+
Double Cheese and Corn Quesadillas	+		+		+	+	+		+	+	+	+
Loaded Moz-zarella Grilled Cheese	+				+	+	+	+	+	+	+	+
Vegetable Pita Pizzas	+		+		+				+		+	+
Lemony Chick-peas with Parsley	+		+		+		+	+			+	

	Lack of Appetite	Nausea, Vomiting, or Heartburn	Constipation	Diarrhea	Fatigue	Mouth Sores	Dry Mouth	Chewing or Swallowing Difficulty	Taste Aversion—Sweet	Taste Aversion—Sour & Bitter	Lack of Taste	Smells Bother
Chickpea Salad Wraps with Toasted Pumpkin Seeds	+		+		+		+		+		+	+
Hummus and Cucumber Tartine	+		+		+		+		+		+	+
Vegetable Wraps with Edamame Spread	+	+	+	+	+	+	+	+	+	+	+	
Spiced Lentil Burritos	+		+		+		+	+	+		+	
Roasted Vegetable Tostadas	+		+		+		+	+	+		+	
Tacos with Peppery Tomato Simmered Lentils	+		+		+		+	+			+	
Shrimp Salad Sandwiches	+		+	+			+		+		+	
Crunchy Tuna Salad Melt	+		+		+		+	+			+	
Roasted Eggplant Pesto Sandwich	+		+		+	+	+		+	+	+	+

Warm Grains, Noodles & Casseroles

	Lack of Appetite	Nausea, Vomiting, or Heartburn	Constipation	Diarrhea	Fatigue	Mouth Sores	Dry Mouth	Chewing or Swallowing Difficulty	Taste Aversion—Sweet	Taste Aversion—Sour & Bitter	Lack of Taste	Smells Bother
Cheesy Quinoa Poppers with Marinara Dipping Sauce	+	+	+		+	+	+	+	+	+	+	+
Green-Flecked Quinoa Oat Cakes	+	+	+		+	+	+	+	+	+	+	+
Warm Quinoa Bowl with Vegetables and Feta	+	+	+		+	+	+	+	+	+	+	+
Veggie Paella	+		+	+	+		+	+	+	+	+	+
Harvest Studded Squash	+	+	+		+		+	+	+	+	+	+
Paprika Chickpeas over Polenta	+			+			+	+	+	+	+	+
Udon Noodles with Sesame Soy Snap Peas	+		+		+	+	+	+	+	+	+	
Your Way Zucchini Noodles	+	+			+		+	+	+	+	+	+
Sweet Potato and Broccoli Mac and Cheese	+	+	+		+	+	+	+	+	+	+	+
Creamy Grits with Roasted Tomatoes and Sautéed Spinach	+	+	+		+		+	+	+	+	+	+
Fettuccine with Green Alfredo	+	+	+		+		+	+	+	+	+	+
Seitan Marinara Pasta Casserole	+		+	+	+		+	+	+	+	+	+
Linguine Presto with Tomatoes, Basil, and Garlic	+		+		+	+	+	+	+	+	+	+
Whole Wheat Couscous Primavera	+		+		+		+	+	+	+	+	
Broccoli Kale Lasagna	+		+		+		+	+	+	+	+	+
Spinach and Scallion Enchiladas	+		+		+		+	+	+	+	+	+
Walnut-Crusted Spinach and Feta Pie	+	+	+		+	+	+	+	+	+	+	+
Tasty Tofu, Quinoa and, Asparagus Casserole	+	+	+	+	+	+	+	+	+	+	+	+

	Lack of Appetite	Nausea, Vomiting, or Heartburn	Constipation	Diarrhea	Fatigue	Mouth Sores	Dry Mouth	Chewing or Swallowing Difficulty	Taste Aversion—Sweet	Taste Aversion—Sour & Bitter	Lack of Taste	Smells Bother
Cheesy Lentil "Meatballs"	+	+	+	+	+		+	+	+	+	+	+
Eggplant and Kidney Bean "Meatballs"	+	+	+	+	+		+	+	+	+	+	+
Vegetarian Sausage	+	+	+	+	+	+	+	+	+	+	+	+
Black Bean Burgers with Sun-Dried Tomatoes and Cilantro	+	+	+		+		+	+	+	+	+	+
Grilled Beet and Goat Cheese Burgers	+		+	+	+	+	+	+	+	+	+	
Balsamic Portobello Cap Burgers	+		+	+	+		+	+	+		+	+
Southwestern Veggie Burgers with Avocado Cilantro Mayo	+		+		+		+	+	+	+	+	+
Chickpea Flour Pizza Margherita	+	+	+	+	+		+		+	+	+	+
Seitan Teriyaki Lettuce Wraps	+		+		+		+	+			+	+
Tempeh Kebabs with Homemade Barbecue Sauce	+		+		+		+		+	+	+	+
Baked Tofu and Broccoli over Wild Rice	+		+		+	+	+		+	+	+	+
Panfried Tofu and Vegetables over Brown Rice	+		+		+	+	+		+	+	+	
Parchment Paper Steamed Fish and Vegetables	+	+	+	+	+		+	+	+	+	+	+
Greek Grilled Salmon with Tzatziki Sauce	+	+	+	+	+		+	+	+	+	+	
Maitake Mushroom and Tomato Poached Salmon	+		+	+	+		+	+	+	+	+	
Moist and Tender Whole Sea Bass on the Grill	+		+	+	+	+	+	+		+	+	
Chicken Ropa Vieja	+	+	+		+		+	+	+	+	+	+
Cilantro Chicken Fajitas	+		+		+		+	+	+	+	+	+
Turkey and Oat Meat Loaf	+	+	+	+	+		+	+	+	+	+	+

Soups & Stews

	Lack of Appetite	Nausea, Vomiting, or Heartburn	Constipation	Diarrhea	Fatigue	Mouth Sores	Dry Mouth	Chewing or Swallowing Difficulty	Taste Aversion—Sweet	Taste Aversion—Sour & Bitter	Lack of Taste	Smells Bother
Cool Cucumber Avocado Soup	+	+	+	+	+	+	+	+	+	+	+	+
Fruit Lovers' Gazpacho	+		+		+		+	+	+	+	+	+
Great Greens Spinach and Kale Soup	+	+	+		+	+	+	+	+	+	+	+
Tuscan White Bean Vegetable Stew	+	+	+	+	+	+	+	+	+	+	+	+
Hearty Tomato Lentil Soup	+		+	+	+		+	+	+	+	+	+
Orzo Kale Soup	+	+	+		+		+	+	+	+	+	+
Carrot Ginger Soup with Cashew Cream	+	+	+		+	+	+	+	+	+	+	+
Simple Mushroom Soup	+	+	+	+	+	+	+	+	+	+	+	+
Asparagus Potato Curry	+		+		+		+	+	+	+	+	+
Spiced and Simmered Green Lentils	+		+		+	+	+	+	+	+	+	+
Sweet Potatoes with Red Lentils and Coconut	+	+	+	+	+	+	+	+	+	+	+	+
Veggie Loaded 3-Bean Chili	+	+	+		+		+	+	+	+	+	+
Sweet Potato Black Bean Chili	+	+	+	+	+		+	+	+	+	+	+
Vegetable Chicken Soup	+	+	+	+	+	+	+	+		+	+	+

	Lack of Appetite	Nausea, Vomiting, or Heartburn	Constipation	Diarrhea	Fatigue	Mouth Sores	Dry Mouth	Chewing or Swallowing Difficulty	Taste Aversion—Sweet	Taste Aversion—Sour & Bitter	Lack of Taste	Smells Bother
Baked Parmesan Swiss Chard Chips	+	+	+		+		+		+	+	+	+
Cinnamon Pear Chips	+	+	+	+	+	+	+			+	+	+
Cranberry Date Chocolate Granola Bites	+		+		+			+		+	+	+
Roasted Applesauce	+	+	+	+	+	+	+	+		+	+	+
Whole Wheat Chocolate Raisin Zucchini Bread	+	+	+		+	+		+		+	+	+
Peaches and Cream Oat Smoothie	+	+	+	+	+	+	+	+		+	+	+
Avocado Mango Smoothie	+	+	+		+	+	+	+		+	+	+
Blueberry Green Nut Butter Smoothie	+	+	+	+	+	+	+	+		+	+	+
Sweet Banana Date Oat Shake	+	+	+	+	+	+	+	+		+	+	+
Blueberry Ginger Coconut Smoothie	+	+	+	+	+	+	+	+		+	+	+
Raspberry Kiwi Julep Smoothie	+	+	+		+	+	+	+	+	+	+	+
Vanilla Almond Chia Seed Shake	+	+	+		+	+	+	+		+	+	+

	Lack of Appetite	Nausea, Vomiting, or Heartburn	Constipation	Diarrhea	Fatigue	Mouth Sores	Dry Mouth	Chewing or Swallowing Difficulty	Taste Aversion—Sweet	Taste Aversion—Sour & Bitter	Lack of Taste	Smells Bother
Carrot Puree with Cilantro Oil	+	+	+	+	+	+	+	+	+	+	+	+
Okra and Corn Succotash	+		+		+		+	+	+	+	+	+
Zucchini Leek Latkes	+	+	+	+	+	+	+	+	+	+	+	+
Asian Stir-Fry with Bok Choy and Mushrooms	+		+		+		+	+	+	+	+	+
Glazed Brussels Sprouts Sauté	+		+		+	+	+	+	+	+	+	+
Cauliflower and Edamame "Rice"	+	+	+		+	+	+	+	+	+	+	+
Hint of Cardamom Spinach Gratin	+		+		+	+	+	+	+	+	+	+
Baked Eggplant Fries with Marinara Dipping Sauce	+		+		+	+	+	+	+	+	+	+
Sautéed Asparagus and Peas	+		+		+	+	+	+	+	+	+	+
Versatile Ratatouille	+		+		+		+	+	+	+	+	
Roasted Roots with Nutmeg Gremolata	+		+		+		+		+	+	+	+
Sautéed Vegetable Medley	+		+		+		+	+	+	+	+	+
Rosemary Vegetables en Papillote	+		+		+	+	+	+	+	+	+	+
Sweet Potato Home Fries	+	+	+	+	+	+	+	+		+	+	+

	Lack of Appetite	Nausea, Vomiting, or Heartburn	Constipation	Diarrhea	Fatigue	Mouth Sores	Dry Mouth	Chewing or Swallowing Difficulty	Taste Aversion—Sweet	Taste Aversion—Sour & Bitter	Lack of Taste	Smells Bother
Peanut Butter Chocolate Banana Whip	+	+	+	+	+	+	+	+		+	+	+
Fudgy Date and Almond Truffles	+	+	+		+	+		+		+	+	+
Cinnamon Honey Baked Bananas	+	+	+	+	+	+	+	+		+	+	+
Frozen Banana Strawberry Bowls	+	+	+	+	+	+	+	+		+	+	+
Molten Dark Chocolate Cake	+		+	+	+	+	+	+		+	+	+
Mini Ricotta Coconut Fruit Pies with Hazelnut Crust	+	+	+		+		+	+		+	+	+
Secret Ingredient Chocolate Banana Pudding	+	+	+	+	+	+	+	+		+	+	+
Dark Chocolate–Coated PB & B Truffles	+		+		+	+	+	+		+	+	+
Chocolate Avocado Fudgsicles	+	+	+	+	+	+	+	+		+	+	+
Chocolate Raspberry Pudding	+	+	+		+	+	+	+		+	+	+
Creamy Coconut Popsicles	+	+	+	+	+	+	+	+		+	+	+
Dark Chocolate Raisin Oat Flour Cookies	+	+	+	+	+			+		+	+	+
Whipped Sweet Potato Pie	+	+	+	+	+	+	+	+	+	+	+	+
Ginger Granita	+	+	+	+			+	+	+	+	+	+
Juicy Grilled Summer Peaches	+	+	+	+	+	+	+	+	+		+	+

Staple Sauces & Condiments

	Lack of Appetite	Nausea, Vomiting, or Heartburn	Constipation	Diarrhea	Fatigue	Mouth Sores	Dry Mouth	Chewing or Swallowing Difficulty	Taste Aversion—Sweet	Taste Aversion—Sour & Bitter	Lack of Taste	Smells Bother
Tomato Habanero Salsa	+		+		+			+	+	+	+	+
Pineapple Mango Salsa	+		+		+		+	+			+	+
Yogurt Hollandaise Sauce	+	+	+	+	+	+	+	+	+	+	+	+
Cucumber Tzatziki	+	+	+	+	+	+	+	+	+		+	+
Aromatic Vegetable Stock	+	+	+	+	+	+	+	+	+	+	+	+
Mirepoix Marinara Sauce	+		+	+	+		+	+	+	+	+	+
Kale Pesto	+		+		+		+	+	+	+	+	+
Basic Pesto	+		+		+		+	+	+	+	+	+
Dijon Balsamic Dressing	+		+		+		+	+	+		+	+
Mediterranean Artichoke Olive Sauce	+		+		+		+	+			+	
Cashew Cream	+		+		+	+		+				+
Supersmooth Ginger Hummus	+	+	+	+	+		+	+	+	+	+	+
Coconut Curry Sauce	+		+		+			+			+	+
Tofu Ricotta	+	+	+	+	+	+	+	+	+	+	+	+

Top Recipes by Symptom

LACK OF APPETITE

Recipe Name	Chapter
Maple Berry Breakfast Parfait	Sweet Mornings
Peach Cardamom Honeyed Yogurt	Sweet Mornings
Eggless Banana Battered French Toast	Sweet Mornings
Classic Avocado Toast	Savory Breakfast & Brunch
Eggy Quinoa Patties	Savory Breakfast & Brunch
Chicken, Apple, and Maple Breakfast Patties	Savory Breakfast & Brunch
Creamy Avocado Egg Salad	Grain Bowls, Salads & Sandwiches
Double Cheese and Corn Quesadillas	Grain Bowls, Salads & Sandwiches
Crunchy Tuna Salad Melt	Grain Bowls, Salads & Sandwiches
Cheesy Quinoa Poppers with Marinara Dipping Sauce	Warm Grains, Noodles & Casseroles
Fettuccine with Green Alfredo	Warm Grains, Noodles & Casseroles
Sweet Potato and Broccoli Mac and Cheese	Warm Grains, Noodles & Casseroles
Cheesy Lentil "Meatballs"	Entrées & Mains
Southwestern Veggie Burgers with Avocado Cilantro Mayo	Entrées & Mains
Chickpea Flour Pizza Margherita	Entrées & Mains
Fruit Lovers' Gazpacho	Soups & Stews
Carrot Ginger Soup with Cashew Cream	Soups & Stews
Veggie Loaded 3-Bean Chili	Soups & Stews
Whole Wheat Chocolate Raisin Zucchini Bread	Snacks & Smoothies
Blueberry Green Nut Butter Smoothie	Snacks & Smoothies
Vanilla Almond Chia Seed Shake	Snacks & Smoothies
Okra and Corn Succotash	Hearty Sides
Hint of Cardamom Spinach Gratin	Hearty Sides
Roasted Roots with Nutmeg Gremolata	Hearty Sides
Peanut Butter Chocolate Banana Whip	Sweet Treats
Fudgy Date and Almond Truffles	Sweet Treats
Mini Ricotta Coconut Fruit Pies with Hazelnut Crust	Sweet Treats
Pineapple Mango Salsa	Staple Sauces & Condiments
Yogurt Hollandaise Sauce	Staple Sauces & Condiments
Supersmooth Ginger Hummus	Staple Sauces & Condiments

NAUSEA, VOMITING, OR HEARTBURN

Recipe Name	Chapter
Apple Crumble Baked Oatmeal	Sweet Mornings
Quinoa Coconut Pancakes	Sweet Mornings
Cinnamon Whole Wheat Waffles	Sweet Mornings
Classic Avocado Toast	Savory Breakfast & Brunch
Eggy Quinoa Patties	Savory Breakfast & Brunch
Chicken, Apple, and Maple Breakfast Patties	Savory Breakfast & Brunch
Chicken Salad with Celery and Grapes	Grain Bowls, Salads & Sandwiches
Vegetable Wraps with Edamame Spread	Grain Bowls, Salads & Sandwiches
Quinoa Bowl with Sliced Avocado and Yogurt Dressing	Grain Bowls, Salads & Sandwiches
Harvest Studded Squash	Warm Grains, Noodles & Casseroles
Creamy Grits with Roasted Tomatoes and Sautéed Spinach	Warm Grains, Noodles & Casseroles
Walnut-Crusted Spinach and Feta Pie	Warm Grains, Noodles & Casseroles
Eggplant and Kidney Bean "Meatballs"	Entrées & Main
Black Bean Burgers with Sun-Dried Tomatoes and Cilantro	Entrées & Main
Chickpea Flour Pizza Margherita	Entrées & Main
Carrot Ginger Soup with Cashew Cream	Soups & Stews
Orzo Kale Soup	Soups & Stews
Vegetable Chicken Soup	Soups & Stews
Baked Parmesan Swiss Chard Chips	Snacks & Smoothies
Sweet Banana Date Oat Shake	Snacks & Smoothies
Blueberry Ginger Coconut Smoothie	Snacks & Smoothies
Zucchini Leek Latkes	Hearty Sides
Cauliflower and Edamame "Rice"	Hearty Sides
Sweet Potato Home Fries	Hearty Sides
Mini Ricotta Coconut Fruit Pies with Hazelnut Crust	Sweet Treats
Creamy Coconut Popsicles	Sweet Treats
Ginger Granita	Sweet Treats
Yogurt Hollandaise Sauce	Staple Sauces & Condiments
Aromatic Vegetable Stock	Staple Sauces & Condiments
Tofu Ricotta	Staple Sauces & Condiments

CONSTIPATION

Recipe Name	Chapter
Raw Blended Buckwheat and Chia Porridge with Raspberries, Apples, and Kiwi	Sweet Mornings
Berry Banana Nut Butter Bowl	Sweet Mornings
Multi-Bran Sour Cream Muffins	Sweet Mornings
Easy-Bake Grab-and-Go Veggie Egg Muffins	Savory Breakfast & Brunch
Sweet Potato, Tomato, and Spinach Hash	Savory Breakfast & Brunch
Seitan, Apple, and Broccoli Breakfast Hash	Savory Breakfast & Brunch
Very Veggie Farro Salad	Grain Bowls, Salads & Sandwiches
Thai Style Vegetable Strand Salad	Grain Bowls, Salads & Sandwiches
Vegetable Pita Pizzas	Grain Bowls, Salads & Sandwiches
Your Way Zucchini Noodles	Warm Grains, Noodles & Casseroles
Broccoli Kale Lasagna	Warm Grains, Noodles & Casseroles
Whole Wheat Couscous Primavera	Warm Grains, Noodles & Casseroles
Southwestern Veggie Burgers with Avocado Cilantro Mayo	Entrées & Mains
Tempeh Kebabs with Homemade Barbecue Sauce	Entrées & Mains
Baked Tofu and Broccoli over Wild Rice	Entrées & Mains
Great Greens Spinach and Kale Soup	Soups & Stews
Hearty Tomato Lentil Soup	Soups & Stews
Spiced and Simmered Green Lentils	Soups & Stews
Baked Parmesan Swiss Chard Chips	Snacks & Smoothies
Whole Wheat Chocolate Raisin Zucchini Bread	Snacks & Smoothies
Avocado Mango Smoothie	Snacks & Smoothies
Cauliflower and Edamame "Rice"	Hearty Sides
Versatile Ratatouille	Hearty Sides
Sautéed Vegetable Medley	Hearty Sides
Frozen Banana Strawberry Bowls	Sweet Treats
Dark Chocolate–Coated PB & B Truffles	Sweet Treats
Juicy Grilled Summer Peaches	Sweet Treats
Pineapple Mango Salsa	Staple Sauces & Condiments
Kale Pesto	Staple Sauces & Condiments
Mediterranean Artichoke Olive Sauce	Staple Sauces & Condiments

DIARRHEA

Recipe Name	Chapter
Sweet Baked Banana Oatmeal	Sweet Mornings
Simple Amaranth Porridge	Sweet Mornings
Cinnamon Whole Wheat Waffles	Sweet Mornings
Classic Avocado Toast	Savory Breakfast & Brunch
Bull's-Eye Skillet Avocado Eggs	Savory Breakfast & Brunch
Sweet or Savory Matzoh Brei	Savory Breakfast & Brunch
Creamy Avocado Egg Salad	Grain Bowls, Salads & Sandwiches
Vegetable Wraps with Edamame Spread	Grain Bowls, Salads & Sandwiches
Shrimp Salad Sandwiches	Grain Bowls, Salads & Sandwiches
Veggie Paella	Warm Grains, Noodles & Casseroles
Paprika Chickpeas over Polenta	Warm Grains, Noodles & Casseroles
Seitan Marinara Pasta Casserole	Warm Grains, Noodles & Casseroles
Balsamic Portobello Cap Burgers	Entrées & Mains
Turkey and Oat Meat Loaf	Entrées & Mains
Greek Grilled Salmon with Tzatziki Sauce	Entrées & Mains
Hearty Tomato Lentil Soup	Soups & Stews
Sweet Potato Black Bean Chili	Soups & Stews
Vegetable Chicken Soup	Soups & Stews
Cinnamon Pear Chips	Snacks & Smoothies
Peaches and Cream Oat Smoothie	Snacks & Smoothies
Sweet Banana Date Oat Shake	Snacks & Smoothies
Carrot Puree with Cilantro Oil	Hearty Sides
Zucchini Leek Latkes	Hearty Sides
Sweet Potato Home Fries	Hearty Sides
Cinnamon Honey Baked Bananas	Sweet Treats
Frozen Banana Strawberry Bowls	Sweet Treats
Dark Chocolate Raisin Oat Flour Cookies	Sweet Treats
Cucumber Tzatziki	Staple Sauces & Condiments
Mirepoix Marinara Sauce	Staple Sauces & Condiments
Tofu Ricotta	Staple Sauces & Condiments

FATIGUE

Recipe Name	Chapter
AB & B Oats	Sweet Mornings
Maple Berry Breakfast Parfait	Sweet Mornings
Multi-Bran Sour Cream Muffins	Sweet Mornings
Bull's-Eye Skillet Avocado Eggs	Savory Breakfast & Brunch
Sweet Potato, Tomato, and Spinach Hash	Savory Breakfast & Brunch
Vegan Mushroom Breakfast Burritos	Savory Breakfast & Brunch
Summery Black Bean, Jicama, and Corn Salad	Grain Bowls, Salads & Sandwiches
Loaded Mozzarella Grilled Cheese	Grain Bowls, Salads & Sandwiches
Hummus and Cucumber Tartine	Grain Bowls, Salads & Sandwiches
Paprika Chickpeas over Polenta	Warm Grains, Noodles & Casseroles
Linguine Presto with Tomatoes, Basil, and Garlic	Warm Grains, Noodles & Casseroles
Spinach and Scallion Enchiladas	Warm Grains, Noodles & Casseroles
Grilled Beet and Goat Cheese Burgers	Entrées & Mains
Panfried Tofu and Vegetables over Brown Rice	Entrées & Mains
Parchment Paper Steamed Fish and Vegetables	Entrées & Mains
Tuscan White Bean Vegetable Stew	Soups & Stews
Asparagus Potato Curry	Soups & Stews
Veggie Loaded 3-Bean Chili	Soups & Stews
Cranberry Date Chocolate Granola Bites	Snacks & Smoothies
Avocado Mango Smoothie	Snacks & Smoothies
Vanilla Almond Chia Seed Shake	Snacks & Smoothies
Asian Stir-Fry with Bok Choy and Mushrooms	Hearty Sides
Sautéed Asparagus and Peas	Hearty Sides
Roasted Roots with Nutmeg Gremolata	Hearty Sides
Juicy Grilled Summer Peaches	Sweet Treats
Secret Ingredient Chocolate Banana Pudding	Sweet Treats
Whipped Sweet Potato Pie	Sweet Treats
Pineapple Mango Salsa	Staple Sauces & Condiments
Basic Pesto	Staple Sauces & Condiments
Super Smooth Ginger Hummus	Staple Sauces & Condiments

MOUTH SORES

Recipe Name	Chapter
AB & B Oats	Sweet Mornings
Simple Amaranth Porridge	Sweet Mornings
Multi-Bran Sour Cream Muffins	Sweet Mornings
Easy-Bake Grab-and-Go Veggie Egg Muffins	Savory Breakfast & Brunch
Sweet or Savory Matzoh Brei	Savory Breakfast & Brunch
Vegan Mushroom Breakfast Burritos	Savory Breakfast & Brunch
Creamy Avocado Egg Salad	Grain Bowls, Salads & Sandwiches
Double Cheese and Corn Quesadillas	Grain Bowls, Salads & Sandwiches
Roasted Eggplant Pesto Sandwich	Grain Bowls, Salads & Sandwiches
Udon Noodles with Sesame Soy Snap Peas	Warm Grains, Noodles & Casseroles
Sweet Potato and Broccoli Mac and Cheese	Warm Grains, Noodles & Casseroles
Tasty Tofu, Quinoa, and Asparagus Casserole	Warm Grains, Noodles & Casseroles
Grilled Beet and Goat Cheese Burgers	Entrées & Mains
Panfried Tofu and Vegetables over Brown Rice	Entrées & Mains
Moist and Tender Whole Sea Bass on the Grill	Entrées & Mains
Cool Cucumber Avocado Soup	Soups & Stews
Great Greens Spinach and Kale Soup	Soups & Stews
Simple Mushroom Soup	Soups & Stews
Roasted Applesauce	Snacks & Smoothies
Whole Wheat Chocolate Raisin Zucchini Bread	Snacks & Smoothies
Blueberry Green Nut Butter Smoothie	Snacks & Smoothies
Glazed Brussels Sprouts Sauté	Hearty Sides
Sautéed Asparagus and Peas	Hearty Sides
Rosemary Vegetables en Papillote	Hearty Sides
Cinnamon Honey Baked Bananas	Sweet Treats
Secret Ingredient Chocolate Banana Pudding	Sweet Treats
Chocolate Avocado Fudgsicles	Sweet Treats
Cucumber Tzatziki	Staple Sauces & Condiments
Cashew Cream	Staple Sauces & Condiments
Tofu Ricotta	Staple Sauces & Condiments

DRY MOUTH

Recipe Name	Chapter
Raw Blended Buckwheat and Chia Porridge with Raspberries, Apples, and Kiwi	Sweet Mornings
Berry Banana Nut Butter Bowl	Sweet Mornings
Apple Butternut Squash Yogurt Pancakesl	Sweet Mornings
Bull'e-Eye Skillet Avocado Eggs	Savory Breakfast & Brunch
Roasted Breakfast Potatoes with Tofu Egg Scramble	Savory Breakfast & Brunch
Cauliflower Crust Quiche	Savory Breakfast & Brunch
Warm Lima Bean and Asparagus Salad with Arugula Parsley Pesto	Grain Bowls, Salads & Sandwiches
Tacos with Peppery Tomato Simmered Lentils	Grain Bowls, Salads & Sandwiches
Crunchy Tuna Salad Melt	Grain Bowls, Salads & Sandwiches
Veggie Paella	Warm Grains, Noodles & Casseroles
Creamy Grits with Roasted Tomatoes and Sautéed Spinach	Warm Grains, Noodles & Casseroles
Broccoli Kale Lasagna	Warm Grains, Noodles & Casseroles
Seitan Teriyaki Lettuce Wraps	Entrées & Mains
Greek Grilled Salmon with Tzatziki Sauce	Entrées & Mains
Turkey and Oat Meat Loaf	Entrées & Mains
Great Greens Spinach and Kale Soup	Soups & Stews
Simple Mushroom Soup	Soups & Stews
Spiced and Simmered Green Lentils	Soups & Stews
Peaches and Cream Oat Smoothie	Snacks & Smoothies
Roasted Applesauce	Snacks & Smoothies
Raspberry Kiwi Julep Smoothie	Snacks & Smoothies
Carrot Puree with Cilantro Oil	Hearty Sides
Baked Eggplant Fries with Marinara Dipping Sauce	Hearty Sides
Versatile Ratatouille	Hearty Sides
Mini Ricotta Coconut Fruit Pies with Hazelnut Crust	Sweet Treats
Chocolate Avocado Fudgsicles	Sweet Treats
Creamy Coconut Popsicles	Sweet Treats
Aromatic Vegetable Stock	Staple Sauces & Condiments
Dijon Balsamic Dressing	Staple Sauces & Condiments
Cashew Cream	Staple Sauces & Condiments

Recipe Name	Chapter
AB & B Oats	Sweet Mornings
Peach Cardamom Honeyed Yogurt	Sweet Mornings
Pineapple and Papaya "Brûlée"	Sweet Mornings
Speedy Spinach Breakfast Tacos	Savory Breakfast & Brunch
Cauliflower Crust Quiche	Savory Breakfast & Brunch
Tofu Scramble with Pesto and Roasted Cherry Tomatoes	Savory Breakfast & Brunch
Lemony Chickpeas with Parsley	Grain Bowls, Salads & Sandwiches
Quinoa Bowl with Sliced Avocado and Yogurt Dressing	Grain Bowls, Salads & Sandwiches
Spiced Lentil Burritos	Grain Bowls, Salads & Sandwiches
Fettuccine with Green Alfredo	Warm Grains, Noodles & Casseroles
Walnut-Crusted Spinach and Feta Pie	Warm Grains, Noodles & Casseroles
Tasty Tofu, Quinoa, and Asparagus Casserole	Warm Grains, Noodles & Casseroles
Cheesy Lentil "Meatballs"	Entrées & Mains
Eggplant and Kidney Bean "Meatballs"	Entrées & Mains
Parchment Paper Steamed Fish and Vegetables	Entrées & Mains
Cool Cucumber Avocado Soup	Soups & Stews
Tuscan White Bean Vegetable Stew	Soups & Stews
Sweet Potato Black Bean Chili	Soups & Stews
Roasted Applesauce	Snacks & Smoothies
Avocado Mango Smoothie	Snacks & Smoothies
Sweet Banana Date Oat Shake	Snacks & Smoothies
Carrot Puree with Cilantro Oil	Hearty Sides
Zucchini Leek Latkes	Hearty Sides
Hint of Cardamom Spinach Gratin	Hearty Sides
Cinnamon Honey Baked Bananas	Sweet Treats
Chocolate Raspberry Pudding	Sweet Treats
Whipped Sweet Potato Pie	Sweet Treats
Tomato Habanero Salsa	Staple Sauces & Condiments
Basic Pesto	Staple Sauces & Condiments
Coconut Curry Sauce	Staple Sauces & Condiments

TASTE AVERSION–SWEET

Recipe Name	Chapter
Pineapple and Papaya "Brûlée"	Sweet Mornings
Apple Butternut Squash Yogurt Pancakes	Sweet Mornings
Multi-Bran Sour Cream Muffins	Sweet Mornings
Easy-Bake Grab-and-Go Veggie Egg Muffins	Savory Breakfast & Brunch
Roasted Breakfast Potatoes with Tofu Egg Scramble	Savory Breakfast & Brunch
Cracked Eggs in Zucchini-Corn-Lime Sauté	Savory Breakfast & Brunch
Quinoa Bowl with Sliced Avocado and Yogurt Dressing	Grain Bowls, Salads & Sandwiches
Very Veggie Farro Salad	Grain Bowls, Salads & Sandwiches
Lemony Chickpeas with Parsley	Grain Bowls, Salads & Sandwiches
Cheesy Quinoa Poppers with Marinara Dipping Sauce	Warm Grains, Noodles & Casseroles
Your Way Zucchini Noodles	Warm Grains, Noodles & Casseroles
Spinach and Scallion Enchiladas	Warm Grains, Noodles & Casseroles
Vegetarian Sausage	Entrées & Mains
Maitake Mushroom and Tomato Poached Salmon	Entrées & Mains
Chicken Ropa Vieja	Entrées & Mains
Tuscan White Bean Vegetable Stew	Soups & Stews
Orzo Kale Soup	Soups & Stews
Veggie Loaded 3-Bean Chili	Soups & Stews
Baked Parmesan Swiss Chard Chips	Snacks & Smoothies
Raspberry Kiwi Julep Smoothie	Snacks & Smoothies
Cinnamon Pear Chips	Snacks & Smoothies
Zucchini Leek Latkes	Hearty Sides
Baked Eggplant Fries with Marinara Dipping Sauce	Hearty Sides
Roasted Roots with Gremolata	Hearty Sides
Whipped Sweet Potato Pie	Sweet Treats
Juicy Grilled Summer Peaches	Sweet Treats
Ginger Granita	Sweet Treats
Cucumber Tzatziki	Staple Sauces & Condiments
Dijon Balsamic Dressing	Staple Sauces & Condiments
Mediterranean Artichoke Olive Sauce	Staple Sauces & Condiments

TASTE AVERSION-SOUR BITTER

Recipe Name	Chapter
Sweet Baked Banana Oatmeal	Sweet Mornings
Eggless Banana Battered French Toast	Sweet Mornings
Maple Berry Breakfast Parfait	Sweet Mornings
Red and Green Eggs Florentine	Savory Breakfast & Brunch
Chicken, Apple, and Maple Breakfast Patties	Savory Breakfast & Brunch
Sweet Potato, Tomato, and Spinach Hash	Savory Breakfast & Brunch
Carrot, Date, and Chickpea Salad	Grain Bowls, Salads & Sandwiches
Chicken Salad with Celery and Grapes	Grain Bowls, Salads & Sandwiches
Loaded Mozzarella Grilled Cheese	Grain Bowls, Salads & Sandwiches
Green-Flecked Quinoa Oat Cakes	Warm Grains, Noodles & Casseroles
Harvest Studded Squash	Warm Grains, Noodles & Casseroles
Linguine Presto with Tomatoes, Basil, and Garlic	Warm Grains, Noodles & Casseroles
Vegetarian Sausage	Entrées & Mains
Tempeh Kebabs with Homemade Barbecue Sauce	Entrées & Mains
Cilantro Chicken Fajitas	Entrées & Mains
Cool Cucumber Avocado Soup	Soups & Stews
Spiced and Simmered Green Lentils	Soups & Stews
Sweet Potatoes with Red Lentils and Coconut	Soups & Stews
Cinnamon Pear Chips	Snacks & Smoothies
Cranberry Date Chocolate Granola Bites	Snacks & Smoothies
Blueberry Ginger Coconut Smoothie	Snacks & Smoothies
Asian Stir-Fry with Bok Choy and Mushrooms	Hearty Sides
Sautéed Asparagus and Peas	Hearty Sides
Sautéed Vegetable Medley	Hearty Sides
Peanut Butter Chocolate Banana Whip	Sweet Treats
Molten Dark Chocolate Cake	Sweet Treats
Mini Ricotta Coconut Fruit Pies with Hazelnut Crust	Sweet Treats
Aromatic Vegetable Stock	Staple Sauces & Condiments
Kale Pesto	Staple Sauces & Condiments
Supersmooth Ginger Hummus	Staple Sauces & Condiments

LACK OF TASTE

Recipe Name	Chapter
Apple Crumble Baked Oatmeal	Sweet Mornings
Sweet Baked Banana Oatmeal	Sweet Mornings
Raw Blended Buckwheat and Chia Porridge with Raspberries, Apples, and Kiwi	Sweet Mornings
Speedy Spinach Breakfast Tacos	Savory Breakfast & Brunch
Cracked Eggs in Zucchini-Corn-Lime Sauté	Savory Breakfast & Brunch
Tofu Scramble with Pesto and Roasted Cherry Tomatoes	Savory Breakfast & Brunch
Warm Lima Bean and Asparagus Salad with Arugula Parsley Pesto	Grain Bowls, Salads & Sandwiches
Spiced Lentil Burritos	Grain Bowls, Salads & Sandwiches
Tacos with Peppery Tomato Simmered Lentils	Grain Bowls, Salads & Sandwiches
Warm Quinoa Bowl with Vegetables and Feta	Warm Grains, Noodles & Casseroles
Veggie Paella	Warm Grains, Noodles & Casseroles
Udon Noodles with Sesame Soy Snap Peas	Warm Grains, Noodles & Casseroles
Black Bean Burgers with Sun-Dried Tomatoes and Cilantro	Entrées & Mains
Balsamic Portobello Cap Burgers	Entrées & Mains
Cilantro Chicken Fajitas	Entrées & Mains
Fruit Lovers' Gazpacho	Soups & Stews
Asparagus Potato Curry	Soups & Stews
Sweet Potatoes with Red Lentils and Coconut	Soups & Stews
Cranberry Date Chocolate Granola Bites	Snacks & Smoothies
Blueberry Green Nut Butter Smoothie	Snacks & Smoothies
Raspberry Kiwi Julep Smoothie	Snacks & Smoothies
Asian Stir-Fry with Bok Choy and Mushrooms	Hearty Sides
Glazed Brussels Sprouts Sauté	Hearty Sides
Rosemary Vegetables en Papillote	Hearty Sides
Fudgy Date and Almond Truffles	Sweet Treats
Chocolate Raspberry Pudding	Sweet Treats
Ginger Granita	Sweet Treats
Tomato Habanero Salsa	Staple Sauces & Condiments
Basic Pesto	Staple Sauces & Condiments
Coconut Curry Sauce	Staple Sauces & Condiments

SMELLS BOTHER

Recipe Name	Chapter
Multi-Bran Sour Cream Muffins	Sweet Mornings
Maple Berry Breakfast Parfait	Sweet Mornings
Quinoa Coconut Pancakes	Sweet Mornings
Red and Green Eggs Florentine	Savory Breakfast & Brunch
Sweet or Savory Matzoh Brei	Savory Breakfast & Brunch
Seitan, Apple, and Broccoli Breakfast Hash	Savory Breakfast & Brunch
Thai Style Vegetable Strand Salad	Grain Bowls, Salads & Sandwiches
Vegetable Pita Pizzas	Grain Bowls, Salads & Sandwiches
Hummus and Cucumber Tartine	Grain Bowls, Salads & Sandwiches
Warm Quinoa Bowl with Vegetables and Feta	Warm Grains, Noodles & Casseroles
Your Way Zucchini Noodles	Warm Grains, Noodles & Casseroles
Fettucine with Green Alfredo	Warm Grains, Noodles & Casseroles
Balsamic Portobello Cap Burgers	Entrées & Mains
Baked Tofu and Broccoli over Wild Rice	Entrées & Mains
Parchment Paper Steamed Fish and Vegetables	Entrées & Mains
Fruit Lovers' Gazpacho	Soups & Stews
Hearty Tomato Lentil Soup	Soups & Stews
Vegetable Chicken Soup	Soups & Stews
Cinnamon Pear Chips	Snacks & Smoothies
Peaches and Cream Oat Smoothie	Snacks & Smoothies
Vanilla Almond Chia Seed Shake	Snacks & Smoothies
Okra and Corn Succotash	Hearty Sides
Cauliflower and Edamame "Rice"	Hearty Sides
Sweet Potato Home Fries	Hearty Sides
Frozen Banana Strawberry Bowls	Sweet Treats
Dark Chocolate–Coated PB & B Truffles	Sweet Treats
Dark Chocolate Raisin Oat Flour Cookies	Sweet Treats
Yogurt Hollandaise Sauce	Staple Sauces & Condiments
Kale Pesto	Staple Sauces & Condiments
Dijon Balsamic Dressing	Staple Sauces & Condiments

Acknowledgments

This cookbook has been a labor of love for everyone at Savor Health. It has truly been a team effort—dietitians, nurses, and our amazing interns who join us from some of the best schools in the country to learn about cancer nutrition and the world of a startup company. Everyone contributed in some way—creating recipes, testing recipes, editing, formatting, you name it. Special thanks to the Savor Health oncology registered dietitians, including Angela Hummel, Holly Mills, Maria Varthis, Aimee Shea, Hillary Sachs, Jocelyn Lutkus, Tasha Feilke, and Jessica Pham as well as our oncology registered nurse, Alyson Gould, and two content and social media experts, Corinne Easterling and Aoi Goto. Registered dietitians, expert chefs, and writing wizards Liv Lee and Stephanie Lang—you were invaluable in testing and revising recipes so that they are as delicious as they are, in writing and editing the book, and in styling the photographs for our photographer, Lou Manna, and his assistant extraordinaire, Joan O'Brien. Lastly, our interns: Thank you to Sydney Greene—you took this project and ran with it. Molly Liebeskind and Mimi Scheidt—you helped us get it across the finish line.

Special thanks also to Jane von Mehren, whose patience and brain power have been a true help in this process. We can't thank her enough for bringing this project to life.

Thanks to the entire team at Da Capo who have been so lovely to work with as we "learn the ropes" of book publishing. We couldn't have been in better hands!

Index